FROM MY

SURVIVING AND THRIVING
IN A FAMILY RAVAGED BY GENETIC DISEASE

A MEMOIR
BY
DARCY LEECH

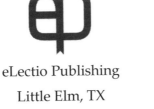

eLectio Publishing

Little Elm, TX

www.eLectioPublishing.com

From My Mother: Surviving and Thriving in a Family Ravaged by Genetic Disease
By Darcy Leech

Copyright 2016 by Darcy Leech. All rights reserved.
Cover design by Darcy Leech and eLectio Publishing. All rights reserved.

ISBN-13: 978-1-63213-224-6
Published by eLectio Publishing, LLC
Little Elm, Texas
http://www.eLectioPublishing.com

Printed in the United States of America

5 4 3 2 1 eLP 20 19 18 17 16

Publisher's Note
The publisher does not have any control over and does not assume any responsibility for author or third-party websites or their content.

Dedicated to Jo Lyn and Dustin Ryan Bartz
May you water the gardens in heaven together.

Author's Note

Some of the individuals who participated in this story asked me to change their names. In the interest of honoring those requests in a way that would not tempt readers to sort out real names from the invented, I chose to alter everyone's name, except for family members. In addition, some details about the location were changed or titles omitted to help preserve privacy.

CONTENTS

Chapter 1
Worth Two Books

I leaned back on a three-foot stuffed polar bear propped against the bedroom wall while reading *Goodnight Moon* to my son, Eli. He was sprawled belly down across his Winnie the Pooh sheets, arm curled under his chin. The soft blue fabric of the blanket my mother made curled along his back, resting just under his bony, pale shoulder.

I read "Goodnight light, and the red balloon" in gentle, soothing words to lull him to sleep. Beneath his close-cut blond hair, his brown eyes scanned for a mouse he knew hid on each page. "Goodnight Bears, Goodnight…"

"There he is!" Eli exclaimed in a nasally toddler voice. His arm shot out, and his short finger pointed to the mouse sitting atop the clothes rack on the page. A dozen baby teeth peeked from his smile, and his wide eager eyes were alert.

"That's right, Eli. There is the mouse. Remember, it's sleepy time." I pursed my lips and gave a mother's look. He snapped his jaw shut and smiled, his youthful dimples below scrunched eyes. Readjusting my shoulders and pushing farther back into the polar bear, I took a deep breath and repeated in a low, calm voice, "Good night Bears, Goodnight Chairs." Eli leaned toward the edge of the bed, inches from the book.

I finished and said, "That's the end of reading tonight," as I flapped the book shut.

His head shot up to shout, "More books, please!", dragging "please" into a widemouthed grin. His smile got me.

"You want more after I read three? I have the book for you." I grabbed *If You Give a Mouse a Cookie*. "This book is about a mouse who asked for more every time he was given something." I made eye contact and paused for emphasis. "Good thing the mouse was in the care of a boy who loved him…" Eli was asleep by page 10.

Watching him sleep reminded me of myself. Smiling, I snuggled farther into the polar bear I always leaned against during reading time, the one that belonged to my mother, the one we had kept in the hospital in her final days. If Eli were like the mouse who asked for more every time he was given something, he came by it honestly. I did the same to my mother. As Eli slept, I reminisced of a time my mother read to me.

My bed, with Strawberry Shortcake sheets and a Care Bear blanket hand sewn by my grandmother, sat under the window. Across the room on the first shelf of my bookshelf sat my collection of Golden Books. My mother, Jo Lyn Bartz, read to me every night she could. We started our night ritual brushing our teeth together. I watched her face behind mine in the mirror; she had long, flowing black hair with wavy curls, pinned back to keep the hair from her eyes. A lock of wavy hair sat in front of her small, well-formed ears. Her cheekbones were high and soft, her lips pouty. Strong dark eyebrows sat evenly and trim above blue eyes that were lighter than mine with gold flecks near the center. We had the same birth mark, a type of stork's bite, with veins in the middle of our forehead that made the track of skin between the top of our nose to the tip of our hair line a slightly darker complexion. My mother was beautiful; fourteen years prior she competed to be Miss Otero County of 1978 as Jo Lyn Woodard.

She noticed I was staring, wrinkled her nose, and stuck out her tongue. I giggled and hunched my shoulders. I stuck my tongue out too and tilted my head in attempt to mimic her expression. At age six, I couldn't scrunch my nose easily. I wanted to; my mother could.

She laid her hand on my shoulder and pointed to the sink, giving the mother look that said more than words. I returned my tongue to its proper place. After finishing, I ran for the bookshelf to find my favorite Golden Book, *Peter Pan*. Perusing the shelf, I found *Ali Baba and the Forty Thieves*. I pondered my options then considered Mother's smile in the mirror. I grabbed both books, snuggled them to my chest, and bolted for the bed, trying to get under the covers before being told to take one back.

Mother walked in and eyed the two books as she sauntered to the chair by my bed. Her slender finger tucked wispy curls behind her ear. She looked at me. I smiled broadly. She reciprocated, but with tight lips. I hadn't noticed the puffy, purple circles under her eyes until I lay in bed. She shifted her weight, grabbed the back of the chair, and sat with stooped shoulders. She sighed audibly. She still had chores.

"Okay, Darcy. I'll read two tonight." Her posture sunk further into the chair. "It's been a long day, but you've been good." Her melodic voice sounded drained as she gazed against the distant white wall. "We haven't had much time together this week," she said without making eye contact. She blinked twice in quick succession. I looked eagerly at her hands around the books. Her nail polish was chipped. Her chest heaved, and she purposefully smiled. With that composed countenance, she turned to face me.

"Let's read."

I soaked in my mother's presence as she read me stories I had heard before but that I heard again because she loved me, because she wanted to spend time with me, because she thought I was worth two books.

***

I wanted to be like my mother; I wanted to invest in reading to my son. I leaned back into the stuffed bear. Mother's favorite animal was a polar bear: she had Coca Cola bears, polar bears on carousels, and a basketful of stuffed polar bears from garage sales. She kept this oversized plush bear, her 'Eli bear,' named after my son, on a guest bed to cuddle. The polar bear was the now in the perfect reading spot next to my son's toddler bed. I'd always valued my mother reading to me, but as a fatigued mother myself, I grasped the magnitude of her exhaustion. That night as a child, I would have had a simple day: school, play, dinner, bed. My mother's day would have been challenging, and she had more to do after story time. Each night she would have gone to bed drained, only to wake up to an oxygen monitor beep two or three times a night. She had more than me to care for; she also had my brother.

Four days before my third birthday, Dustin came into the world. Mom never talked about the week Dustin was born, the emotional syphon of not being near me and unable to hold her infant, or the complications of delivering a boy who would have open heart surgery, a feeding tube, and a ventilator. She didn't have me, her first, until she was twenty-five. Dad shared after I had my first child that Mom had suffered through multiple miscarriages. I was at least the third time my mother had carried a child. In grade school, I would have been told and repeated a banal stock phrase like "My brother was born with congenital myotonic dystrophy, a severe form of muscular dystrophy, the disease Jerry Lewis collects money for on TV. Dustin had to have open heart surgery after birth and spent most of his first three years of life in the hospital." I did not comprehend the complications affecting Mom when I would beg for extra books.

Mom went to the hospital to deliver Dustin three weeks early and underwent an emergency C-Section. Dad heard the doctor say "That is a lot of liquid" as amniotic fluid poured from the incision. The doctor's voice was quick, direct, efficient – not a casual remark. The doctor pulled the baby from the womb, laid him down on the medical tray, and cut his umbilical cord. He was placed in the arms of his father. The baby didn't cry; he barely stirred. Two minutes later, the bluish baby boy was taken from his father without his mother being cognizant enough to notice.

My brother failed to thrive and was taken, attached to life support, on a two hour helicopter flight from Blythville Air Force Base in Arkansas to Tennessee. Seven weeks later, Dustin would be again transported by helicopter to Wilford Hall Ambulatory Surgical Center, a U.S. Air Force medical treatment facility in San Antonio, Texas. Something had gone wrong, something invisible until Dustin's skin turned blue, something genetic - congenital. Mom met Dustin in Texas three days later. Her first conscious sight of her son, he was asleep behind thick glass in an isolation incubator with a four-inch intravenous needle protruding from his skull.

My father, Randy Bartz, was an Air Force Civil Engineer and returned to work after Dustin's birth. Mom lived in Wilford Hall, sleeping in a parent room affiliated with the neonatal intensive care unit near Dustin. Dad kept me in Arkansas. The Air Force worked diligently to change Dad's assignment so we could live as a family near Wilford Hall. I went to meet my brother in a moving truck packed with all our belongings.

I met Dustin when he was three months old. Dad had prepared me with multiple conversations about Dustin's health and why Mom hadn't been home lately. In all my memory, I've known Dustin would die before me; I was told that before I met him.

At the hospital, Dad and I were escorted to a changing room. The nurse pointed to a small blue scrub I'd wear to meet my brother. The front had a black Wilford Hall logo, a snake wrapped around a staff surrounded by lightning. Dad, with a military trained six foot frame and hairy arms, tenderly gathered my hair in a ponytail bun. The nurse made sure no hair protruded from under my hair net.

"Darcy, you need a mask. Our germs might harm Dustin." Dad spoke with massive hands on my quivering shoulders. The nurse slid the mask over my nose and ensured a snug fit. Dad had tried to prepare me for this moment during our ten-hour road trip, but with the unfamiliar cloth restricting my breathing, the snake crest upon my chest – I was terrified. That changing room is vivid in my memory because that is when Dad's conversations about "birth complications" and "disease" became tangible to a preschool girl.

Somehow though, my memories of meeting Dustin are clouded in positive comfort. I've kept a picture of the day I met Dustin:

> *In the picture's center, I sit on Dad's lap. The mask covers my mouth, but my squinted eyes are smiling. The neckline of my too-large blue scrub dips below my sternum, revealing the pink and white stripes of my shirt. The hair net is almost as wide as my shoulders. Dad is dressed in a striped button up shirt with a crisp collar. His yellow disposable smock is too small. His dark brown mustache is freshly trimmed and his hair cut to military regulations. Years of physical training have made his long neck broad and sturdy. Standard thick-rimmed military glasses sit on his nose as he looks towards Dustin's hospital bed. He is*

whispering in my ear. Dad's bulbous knuckles rest on my legs, and even with a snake logo over my heart, I look happy.

Dustin's head dominates his body; his lax, droopy muscles seem to occupy space like baggy clothes on a thin frame. To build lung strength, Dustin received steroid injections. The weight gain clumped in his cheeks. Dustin's high, wide forehead separates deep set brown eyes from his brow, shaved for the recently removed large IV protruding from his head while in the incubator.

An oxygen tube envelopes his face, the tight fit pushing his nose. Dustin's open mouth has a triangular shape as his tongue protrudes slightly, a sign of orofacial dysfunction common in children with myotonic muscular dystrophy.

Atop the rail guard of Dustin's hospital crib, my brother grips my hand with his pale fingers never exposed to the sun. Dad's other hand is behind me, stroking his infant son's head.

In the picture we look happy. We made the best of it. Mother took the picture. She isn't in many pictures or memoires from that era.

While Dad worked, Mom tried to be Dustin's reason to live. She was constantly near Dustin, knew every medical procedure, communicated with staff, sang to him, held his hand, and caressed his face. She was ripped from her home and lived from a suitcase, sleeping in a hospital guest bed. Separated from her husband, without her daughter, rarely seeing her mother or any friends, she relinquished all former social connections, hoping Dustin would live to make his own choices, experience life, live and breathe in a real bedroom, play outdoors, and run to hug her like I could. Jo Lyn did not work while Dustin was in the hospital, go to parties, or sleep next to her husband in their bedroom. She was bound to her son's progress, devoted to giving him a chance at survival.

Dustin came home, but he would make thirteen more ambulance trips and three more helicopter flights to a hospital in the first three years of his life. In addition to open heart surgery shortly after birth,

Dustin had an apnea monitor, oxygen machine, and feeding tube. He spent twice the nights in the hospital as he did at home. Dustin was four when his feeding tube was removed and he began eating baby food.

Most people who experience myotonic muscular dystrophy have symptoms that aren't noticeable until after age thirty – like one man, a retired large company executive who didn't learn he had myotonic muscular dystrophy (MMD) until late middle age. He had been active in sports throughout high school and had a football scholarship in college. He was fifty-four when he began noticing muscle weakness in his hands. "I was trying to clean my glasses," he recalls, "and my thumb couldn't push the spray." He can still enjoy sports like golfing but has a pacemaker and must monitor his activity level and energy.

Many people afflicted with MMD, like my mother, seem normal and are unaware they carry a degenerative muscle disease. One man affected by MMD lived to be seventy-six and was a successful businessman, textbook author, and world traveling travel writer for the national Quest Magazine. A 2012 Quest article by Margaret Wahl portrayed the MMD experience. For example, one woman from Texas remembered how her mother had difficulty opening jars, even when she was in her twenties. It's something a daughter or a doctor might notice, but perhaps no one else. By age seventeen years, she too had issues with her hands "locking up" as well as other symptoms that were similar to those that ultimately led to her mother's death at age fifty-two.

MMD often isn't a problem until adulthood. When MMD begins during adulthood, it can progress slowly. Many with MMD can walk, talk, and live independently. However, MMD varies greatly in severity, sometimes even within the same family.

The type of MMD that begins in adolescence or isn't recognized until adulthood can be drastically different from what affects newborns, congenital MMD. Babies with congenital MMD have severe muscle weakness, including weakness in necessary muscle functions for survival like breathing and swallowing. This muscle weakness is life-threatening, and infants with the congenital form need intensive care. While males born with the adult-onset MMD may live to face early balding and adjust to weakening neck muscles and loss of grip strength, males born with the congenital version experience a higher and more rapid severity of symptoms. Before 1989, when Dustin was born, few infants with congenital MMD survived.

An infant with congenital MMD faces a tough road in getting home from the hospital. In 2009, Susan Jane gave birth to a son with myotonic dystrophy, Lee, in a story similar to my brother's from 1989. "About twelve minutes after he was born, he quit breathing while my husband was holding him," she recalls. Infants like Lee and Dustin struggle to breathe and often do not have the muscle strength to swallow. Lee, like Dustin, was taken swiftly from his parents and to a neonatal intensive care unit and placed on a ventilator before being transferred a week later to a larger hospital for continued care. Even after coming home from a neonatal intensive care unit, an infant with congenital MMD will need a feeding tube and supplemental oxygen to continue the necessary life functions of eating and breathing.

Cases vary, but many children with congenital MMD who do survive the first few years will see an impressive gain in ability. In 2011, at age two, Lee was able to sleep in his own room without oxygen. My brother, Dustin, outgrew the need for nightly oxygen by age eight. Early physical, occupational, and speech therapy can help children with MMD see significant gains. At age two, Lee's vocabulary was limited to 'uh-oh' and 'yee-hah', but he was gaining ability, and the family invested in learning sign language. Dustin learned basic sign language to express his wants, and could form repetitive sounds like 'dadadada.' Now in 2015, an infant with congenital MMD has not only greater chances of survival but also greater assistance in gaining ability and more shared medical knowledge and advocacy in the MMD community.

In 1989, a doctor said Dustin was "one in a million," defying odds by surviving with a genetic intensity of MMD previously unwitnessed at the best military hospital in America. The specialist staff at Wilford Hall believed Dustin's complications were genetic. A specialist who shook my mother's hand and noted her difficulty in returning her hand to its usual position when he released his grip diagnosed her as also carrying MMD shortly after he diagnosed Dustin. Like the woman from Texas, her hand would lock up. I was a healthy girl born to a seemingly healthy mother, but the doctors worried I carried a latent gene that could manifest adult onset symptoms like Mom. In 1989 our family life progressed on the edge of medical knowledge.

Six years after Dustin's birth in 1992, scientists discovered the genetic mutation causing MMD. J. David Brook, a molecular biologist and leader of the groups discovering the genetic link, cautioned "treatment is not just around the corner." Today in 2015, there is still no known cure or long-term preventative treatment. Experimental fields of genetic therapy may hold promise. Science is moving quickly and perhaps some alive today will live to see a cure. Years after Dustin was born, as I sat next to my son's bed, I tried to envision what motherhood was like as the transmitter of a genetic and terminal disease.

Mom's world immutably altered with the birth of her second child, a son with special and immediate needs. Dad's life changed too, but not as precipitously. He was contracted in the Air Force and returned to going to work daily. Everything changed for Mom. She had a tragic birth experience, her body weakened and scarred by the cesarean operation, her emotions gutted as her son was flown across state borders and she was unable to hold him or nurse. Beyond the traumatic stress of delivery and neurological aftermath of postpartum depression, she was ripped from her home, her friends, and waitressing job. Her life was asunder, altered irrevocably by a birth that brought a boy in the world to fight for his every breath and revealed a lingering and dormant genetic harbinger in her own genetic code: adult onset myotonic muscular dystrophy type one. That was just the beginning of her sacrifices.

My eyes lingered on my restful son. His cheek bones protruded like my husband's, a healthy man from a family with no trace of MMD. Eli's body and language abilities seemed to be developing on a pace like mine or his father's. I daydreamed as a young girl of being the parent of a child like my brother. Growing up, I idealized my parents. Mom was a woman of strength, small in build but wise and weathered to withstand any storm, capable to make tough decisions and endure what must be endured. When she was home with me, Mom seemed the bastion of what a woman should be – caring and capable.

Dustin shifted the seismograph of my parents' emotions range, but I didn't comprehend the magnitude. I rarely saw Mom cry, even if I saw her red eyes after she came out from being alone in her bedroom. In imaginative play, my baby dolls were born with muscular dystrophy, but fathoming life from Mom's perspective was beyond what play enabled. At age twenty-eight, reading to my son as my mother read to me, I began to understand. Tears fell in gratitude for Eli's ability to use words to ask for another book, something Dustin never had.

I still have a fear of snakes and despise fabric over my nose. I resented coloring after finishing every page in the book I carted to one hundred waiting rooms in a duffle bag of broken crayons. I had trouble relating to the mother who use to dote on me and was then gone so often or near exhaustion from caring constantly for Dustin. I didn't know how to make the pretty braids in my hair that I saw in pictures of my mother when she was my age. Surviving and thriving in a family ravaged by genetic disease wasn't easy; it took an indomitable optimism, an indefatigable fighter's will, and the intrinsic love of a mother. Next to Eli's bed, I clasped my hands tightly and prayed to God for my son's continued health.

Chapter 2
Wishing

Most my early childhood memories are with my father. Even as I admired Mom, her dedication to Dustin in the hospital meant I didn't see her much. If I went to the hospital, I went with Dad because Mom was already there. If someone gave me a long talk about what Dustin was going through, it was Dad. If I wanted to play at home, I probably played Legos or forts with Dad.

In waiting rooms and cars, Dad talked with me about the nature of life, God's will in disease, why we shouldn't fear death. He told me how lucky I was, and how I could be a blessing to others in the hospital. I became an introverted, serious daddy's girl. To contrast the stark reality of our life so often spent near a hospital, Dad indulged me in a fanciful habit by always stopping at wishing wells. Whatever my grade school brain rationalized about genetics or medicine or superstition, I believed that at wishing wells I could wish my way to a better day.

I was seven, and Dad and I were at a grassy opening with four sidewalks leading to a central water fountain. Creamy white brick hospital buildings surrounded three sides of the clean cut green grass in an outdoor courtyard featuring water that cascaded down three tiers to a brick pool. Dustin was in the hospital, and Mom was by his side. Like enough of my early days, Dad and I were strolling around the hospital campus waiting on the outcome.

Dad's eyes were tired, his shoulders stooped. He spoke to me in a solemn, adult voice about topics from which children are often sheltered, like how easily death could take a loved one. Like Mom, Dustin's birth had separated Dad from his friends. His parents and siblings were all at least two states away. I was Dad's confidant.

Dad's clean shaven face was emotionally ragged, his rumpled old t-shirt thrown on in haste after rushing home. "Darcy, your brother has been a wonderful blessing..." he began in a somber tone. "I've learned so much about being a father in the last few years." He kicked at the ground as he spoke. "You've had to sacrifice so much as a child, play with random kids at parks near the hospital and occupy yourself for hours in waiting rooms."

"I'm pretty good at Super Mario. Most the hospitals have it." I moved my thumbs like I held that Super Nintendo controller and grinned.

His weary eyes looked in mine; his neck craned over with stress. He yearned to be able to grin like his daughter. He gave a short half humored laugh and looked back down at the ground. "Maybe you'll get more time to be a kid -- play Mario at home instead of in hospitals or hotels." He stared off at the outer façade of the hospital where Dustin was. He closed his eyes and sighed. "I haven't been able to be the best father for you and all that. What do you want most? Do you know what it takes for you to be happy?"

From my perspective as a seven-year-old, my brother had only ever gotten stronger. Every time the doctors said Dustin wouldn't make it, he had. Dustin gained vitality every year, and I adamantly believed Dustin would walk and talk. My prayers seemed that they were being answered because I saw Dustin improve and cross new thresholds so often. I believed God would heal my brother. I hadn't lived long enough to see death take anyone, didn't understand science enough to comprehend the challenges, and felt like my prayers and wishes were part of the reason Dustin persisted.

"Can I have a quarter?"

Dad searched my face trying to capture that spark a child's unjaded hope can offer.

"A quarter? That can't buy much. Darcy, I'm serious. I want to be a better dad for you."

"Don't be silly. I want a quarter for the well."

He nodded and pursed his lips in thought. "Hmm…"

He knew what I did not. This time the doctor had said, "It will be a miracle if he makes it." Mom was distraught, thinking this might be the day she lost her son. What would a wishing well do? He drew a weighty breath and let out a beleaguered half-laugh. "Well, what's the harm?" he said as he handed over the quarter.

I slid my hand in his and pulled toward the fountain. My other hand gripped that quarter. When we reached the well, I closed my eyes, tightened my whole body, and felt a shiver travel my spine. My heart burned. I was young and hopeful. Prayers felt so natural. My heart believed quarters cast in water could bring about Dustin's healing. The quarter wedged between my fleshy palms as I prayed in supplication. I brought my hands to my face, stuck my nose between my fingers and breathed. I prayed with the willpower of a young heart that hadn't seen prayer fail. I knew my brother would get better; he always had. With unfettered faith, I prayed until the heat in my chest turned to warm security and cast the quarter into the pool, pushing both hands out from my face. "Amen."

Silence lingered. I opened my eyes. Small ripples waved towards the bricks as the quarter sat on the bottom of the pool. Dad raised his eyes from the water. He was a grown man trained to protect his country; I couldn't tell if I was seeing the reflection of the well or if his own eyes were pooling. His lips crept towards his eyes, but the sad weight in his cheeks held them down. He croaked, "What did you wish for?"

"I asked God to let Dustin walk one day, Daddy. It's what I always wish for."

Dad smiled under his tired eyes. In a conference that day, he heard the doctor's analytical voice drone about possible outcomes. However naïve it may have been, my optimistic voice was a comfort. He hugged me.

After a rocky operation and a few nights on IV drip and constant oxygen, Dustin survived. Mom got to sleep in her own bed, Dad went back to work, I returned to school, and Dustin continued to get stronger.

As a family surviving and thriving with genetic disease, life wasn't always that climatic. We had genial moments when Dustin was in stable health at home. Later that year, 1993, in Texas, the four of us were home together. Dad sat beside Mom on our timeworn yellow floral print couch. Dad, tired from work, sank in against one of the short arms. His large hand encompassed Mom's whole right thigh as they sat hip to hip.

On a blanket in the middle of the living room, Dustin lay next to a toy designed for the early stages of life with a plastic blue base and yellow, red, and blue looping wires that housed colorful beads. His nasal cannula tubes wrapped around his head, dominated his diminutive body, and tethered him to a metal green oxygen tank on wheels. The plastic nozzle for his 'nasogastric intubation', his feeding tube, protruded through his second hand Mickey Mouse shirt, which was wet around the collar with drool. Above his collar, emblazoned on his soft white skin, was a bulging scar of bright pink flesh, that when completely visible, slashed from the tip of his collar bone to his stomach – the keloid scar from his life-saving open heart surgery performed shortly after birth.

Dustin lay on his back with his double jointed legs sprawled without the restrictions of tight hip muscles. His toes curled in, pulling towards his heel like a hook. By age three he could roll over or sit for short periods, but not crawl easily due to his muscle strength and tubing. He rolled over to his side then pushed mightily with his arms to come to a sitting position. He yearned for the beads beyond his grasp. With loose legs in front of him, he tried to reach his upper body forward, lean on one elbow, and grab the beads with the other. When he didn't succeed he moaned in frustration and craned his neck over to me.

I put down my Legos and walked over to Dustin, who watched my approach. I stooped to grab the bead set then sat next to my brother. His face seemed so soft, with loose cheeks hanging with the floppiness of Droopy the cartoon dog. The bead rose up the wire and cascaded down as I spun it with my finger. His chest rose as a hiss of interest escaped between his raised upper lip shaped like a tent, and his loose bottom lip, which hung below his gum line. Bubbles of slobber escaped his mouth. I flicked harder, sending the bead around one full loop and halfway around another. Dustin's chest heaved in pleasure as a throaty chuckle pushed past his mouth. He placed a soft, cushiony hand on the yellow wire and extended his fleshy forefinger, spinning a square cube in place. His eyes brightened in intellectual engagement. His brain was learning. Excited to see him fully engaged, I played with him spinning beads, making noises, hiding the bead set behind his back to reveal it again. His laughter shook his plumpish belly.

I sat the beads just beyond his reach.

"Grab it, Dustin." I stuck my hand out and pinched my fingers together, giving a gesture to match my words. He raised his shoulders and tightened his neck muscles. He understood, but that body posture also meant he anticipated difficulty. He was scared. Conventional stomach crawling wasn't an option for a child with a feeding tube, nor was rolling over multiple times. He didn't want to experience pain to grab the toy. His sat and stared. His eyes were locked on the toy as he processed his options. I sat cross legged on the floor and placed my hands fingers splayed out, palms down on the floor. I waited as he thought.

"Scoot, like this." I bent my elbows and put weight right below my fingers, raising my body enough to use my core muscles to move my legs. Then, I brought my arms forward to about my knees again, resting on one arm to be able to extend the other to pick up the toy and place it down.

Dustin placed his palms on the ground and attempted to lift his body. His arms were flimsy and pliable. I loved to rest my head on his bicep like a pillow while we cuddled. His doughy arms didn't budge him. He flapped both bony knees up and let his limp legs clop on the ground. His calves reshaped to the ground like balloons filled with sand. He grunted again, this time at Dad. Dad patted Mom's leg, pushed to lift his tired body from the couch, and walked behind my brother, kneeling behind Dustin.

"You gotta move your bottom, Udey-dude." Udey-dude was the nickname I gave Dustin after watching Ninja Turtles, 'Udey' for short. Loosening his neck muscles, Dustin let the back of his head touch his spine to see Dad behind him. I tried mimicking the move, my denser muscles nowhere near as flexible as his. Dad waved his fingers in front of Dustin's face then lifted Dustin's head to a normal position.

"Okay. Like this." Dad maneuvered Dustin's hands in front of his legs, helped lean his shoulders forward, then put his own hands wide across the back of Dustin's hips. Dad's hands had tight skin and visible veins. Dustin's looked more like something on a stretch Armstrong toy, as if you could squeeze through to feel your other fingers. Dustin tried again to push with those muscles.

"Now push here." Dad nudged Dustin forward by pushing his hips. My brother, with a wide-open mouth slobbering down a trail of drool, turned to look at Dad behind him, who pointed toward the beads.

Dustin inhaled deeply, processing again. He leaned forward, put his weight on his flabby arms, and pushed his hips to scoot forward. He grabbed the toy. Dustin raised his shoulders and huffed in a show of triumph. Mom clapped and said "Good job, Udey!" Dustin spun the beads as his eyes narrowed in complete focus. Dad smiled and extended to his full kneeling height with a chest puffed in pride.

I sat in awe of Dustin's willpower. For a healthy kid Dustin's age, scooting forward a few inches would be uncelebrated, a waste of time. To our family, this simple success reinforced our progressive hope with tangible results. Despite his tubes and tethers, labels and limitations, this four-year-old boy was learning to get what he wanted and enjoying the process. He didn't recognize what he didn't have or dwell on our capabilities compared against his own. He didn't cry because he couldn't walk to the toy. He just saw the toy, saw a way, and grew. I stood awash in the glow of believing that, by love, willpower, and prayer, Dustin was getting stronger every day.

I was getting stronger too, a capable seven-year-old girl who loved to run, play softball, and ride bikes. Not always content to settle on the blanket with Dustin, I yearned for physical challenge. Some time after the day Dustin learned to scoot, I asked Dad, my usual athletic partner, to join me on a bike ride. A salt ring capped the brown military t-shirt he still wore from work.

"Oh, Darce, I'm too tired, little girl." He stretched his arm out and laid his head back. "I just want to sit here on the couch and watch Dustin play." Randy served the Air Force as a civil engineer in water maintenance, and some days that meant digging ditches, laying pipe, and coming home sore.

I groaned. I had been inside for hours, sat at a desk in school, played rug games on the floor with Dustin, and I'd already dug to the bottom of my toy box for one of last year's favorites. I slouched to the shelf with the coloring books, reached for a book, and then lethargically dropped my hand in defeat.

Mom took the ladle out of the pot and sat the corn heat on low. She sauntered toward the living room and called out: "Dinner's in the oven, hun. If I go for a bike ride, can you take it out with the buzzer?"

I spun to face her. Daily medical maintenance tasks and sleepless nights had changed her body, but she looked like she could still pedal. "Really, Mom? You'd go?" I dashed to grab my helmet.

"You'll have to be patient with me dear; I haven't ridden my bike since before Dustin was born." Mom held her hand on her stomach, fingering over the cesarean scar. We went to the garage. My purple bike rested on its kickstand near the door. An old Huffy road bike with a high seat and cruiser handle bar, Mom's bike had rusty gears and a low tire. After ten minutes of labor, the bikes were out, and her tire was ready.

I tottered in my recent training wheel freedom; Mom wobbled too. Sun light enveloped my arms as the breeze caressed my cheeks. Riding outdoors, alone with Mom, was a rare liberation.

"Mom, this is great! Watch, I can do a figure eight!" I shouted as I peered back at Mom. She peddled in her blue trousers, worn-out tennis shoes, and loose blouse. Hair escaped her pony tail to assail her eyes.

She smiled, her face shining despite haggard breathing. "I didn't know you could do that already! You learn so fast..." Her voice drifted as I finished the figure eight and tried to stand up on the pedals to push hard to climb the incline to the sidewalk. I nearly lost control on the slope, righted myself then kept riding, outpacing my mother.

"Wow! You're marvelous on a bike!" Mom was my biggest fan. "Can you use your --" she began. Her check hung slack, as if she were frowning. She swallowed and started again, "-- use your brakes very well?" Eager to please, I launched forward, turned sharply, then threw my weight against the pedal brakes to leave a tire trail right up to her bike. I beamed, happy to perform as the sole object of her attention.

"How's that? Soon I'll be ready for wheelies! Can we go ride the school black top?"

Her jaw snapped shut. "I...." She frowned. "I don't think we should. I don't want to leave Dustin too long." I looked wistfully toward the park.

I sighed and nodded, "Okay." I indulged in winding turns along the flat road, prolonging the moment I had Mom alone.

Sweat glistened under her stork bite birth mark, which flared red from exertion. Mom's allergies and asthma were agitated by our late spring ride. She labored three more blocks before we headed back. I coasted into the driveway and waited for her to pedal the last half block.

In the driveway, she braked and reached her toes for the cement. Awkwardly, she fell off the seat as her feet came abruptly to the ground. Her pedal jammed against her leg. "Oww!" She dropped the bike and jumped over the frame. I flicked my kickstand and ran to Mom.

"Are you okay?" I asked as I gazed at the pedal spiked gashes on her leg.

She placed her arm on my shoulder and leaned on me. "Oh, I think I will be." She smiled sheepishly as her small round nose scrunched against her cheeks. "I've never been great at riding bikes." She let out an embarrassed laugh. She limped to the house with an awkward gait, leaning heavily on me.

There were differences between me and Mom. I loved softball, bikes, running, and recess football. While Mom had never been athletic, she cheered me on with constant and favorably biased support. I loved much about Mom, but my favorite way to spend time with her was to perform in front of her. She coached my softball team one year with Dad when I was four. While Dad had coached me many more years, Mom transitioned to a spectator who would come to every game, throw awkwardly with me in the yard, and tell me how amazing I was. Mom enabled me to feel capable, confident, and supported. I grew up thinking Mom just wasn't interested in being athletic herself. I missed the implications of what having a brother with a degenerative muscle disease meant for Mom's body, or for our family finances.

Paying the full insurance deductible and coinsurance each year made money tight. The military assigned Dad closer to Wilford Hall, let him take medical emergency time, and guaranteed him a job no matter the costs incurred through hospitals and insurance. The military is why we survived financially. Mom quit her job after Dustin was born. A county program in Texas paid for 20 hours a week of in-house hospice nurse care for Dustin. With a home health care nurse able to watch Dustin during the day, Mom returned to work. Mom wanted to see me more, but she also wanted to try to help ease the family financial bind and feel like she still had a life of her own. We began to chip away at the mounds of medical debt. Mom went back to waitressing during the day and came back to Dustin and me to cook dinner, brush Dustin's teeth, get us ready for bed, and check all the medical equipment. It didn't leave much time for pretend play or bike rides.

Not long after she went back to work, I packed my pillow with supplies and told my mother I was running away. The outward show of our separation wounded her. Distraught, she called the school counsellor. The counsellor probed the psychology of my second-grade mind by asking about my happiness, my home life, and why I would want to run away. In the end, she told me to go home and tell Mom I love her and apologize, to which I obediently, if not warmly complied.

One day after school soon after, Mom and I were painting at the kitchen table. I was enjoying trying to guess the compliments Mom would give my art when instead she asked me to stop to help her with Dustin. He let out a loud grumble of a cry, like the moan of a young walrus. Mom checked his temperature, readjusted his nasal tubes, cleaned around his feeding tube, and checked his diaper. "How are you feeling, Udey? Is it your foot?"

She massaged his curved club feet, which sometimes hurt after being in shoes through the school day. His groans subsided, and his legs lost their tension as he relaxed into the floor, making sure to touch Mom with his leg and to grab her arm.

"Darcy, hold Dustin's hand for me." She changed his diaper. When she finished, she asked me to take the diaper to the outdoor trash can, which I did. I came back into the house eager to finally paint.

"Darcy, can you find the mushrooms in the cupboard?"

I huffed and rummaged through the cupboard.

"Darcy, can you be gentler? We need to keep things organized in there." She called over her shoulder.

I smacked a green bean can hard against another. "I can't find any stupid mushrooms." I crossed my arms and sulked on the floor. "Can't I just go back and paint like any normal kid would? I have to do so much of everybody else's work around here." I raised my voice at her and under a defiant glare stated the obvious. "I'm a kid!"

She eyed me coolly over her shoulder. "Try the second shelf," she said in a flat, even voice. My look of disgust shifted from her to the second shelf.

"There are no mushrooms there either. Find your own mushrooms! I already took out the diaper. Dustin isn't my son!" Her eyes narrowed on me, not in shock or anger but in one of those moments that focus a person on an inconvenient truth.

"You should take better care of what you brought into the world!" I stomped back to the table aggressively and thumped down in my chair as if I had won some emphatic battle challenge. Mom continued cooking, her back turned to me.

She took her time pouring and measuring. After longer than necessary, she came back to sit with me and painted again, head down. She sighed heavily and then sniffled. Her eyes watered.

I felt guilty. After a while, I said "Mom, I'm sorry. I just hate taking out diapers -- and I don't like mushrooms."

She looked at me. Her drained eyes were weary from lack of sleep and a job that kept her on her feet. She rested her cheek on her knuckle. "I just spoke with your teacher at conferences last week. She talked about how nice you were, how you were always polite, and how you helped anyone in your group and knew so many answers." Her voiced wavered. "Mrs. Greene even said you volunteered to hand out papers and always make sure your group area was clean." Guilt welled inside me as I saw the pain in her eyes. I never back-talked my teacher.

"You're so good at school. Your teachers love you." I wished I could escape like the tear dashing down her cheek. When she was emotional, she began to slur her words and speak in a higher pitch. "Why aren't you more of a helper here?" Her voice cracked. She closed her eyes and let the tears fall. I lifted my brush to paint another stroke. Her head slumped into the crevice of her arm. She cried as I sat ashamed, trying to find what to say.

"I don't know, Mom. I don't know. Do I have to help all the time?" I stared at my feet and wiped my runny nose. "... I don't like to cook."

She rose her head again as she tried to smile. "I know you don't, Darcy. I'll try not to ask too much of you." She forced her smile. She had to do that sometimes, give extra effort to make her lips curl up. "I appreciate your help with Dustin. It does make life easier."

She was still slurring her words.

"Yeah, Mom. I know." I made two more strokes and shook my brush out in the water. "Can I be excused? I want to go read."

She let me leave. I looked back at her. Constant angst had worn wrinkles onto her young face. Her eye sockets seemed to dig burrows into her face after she cried. I went to my room and read about characters that flew on magic carpets and escaped to a world of more adventure than chores and where no one sat in a wheelchair.

I could have sat in my room and reflected on the sacrifices Mom made for her two children, or admired her capacity for love and endurance. I could have wondered what she had gone through with Dustin's birth, discovering she had the same disease, knowing it would have an adult onset form waiting for her, then having to work to support the family financially. I didn't. Children rarely think like that. Instead, I sulked on how much work I had to do around the house compared to my friends and escaped to a fictional world of magic and limitless possibilities.

Mom did wonderfully and I'm glad she was patient because my maturation took a while. I fought her. I didn't always like the way she gave me attention. I had more fun pretending to be a world saving hero in a video game than helping with her burdens. I was a typical kid in an atypical situation. However, Mom battled her fear and negativity. She did what needed to be done. Somehow she overcame her pain and the stress of having a child so often on the edge of life to raise me with the abundant resources of love and honest life lessons.

Chapter 3
Salt Lake

"Slow down," Mom called after me as I bounded in long-legged pre-teen strides down the gypsum beach towards the Great Salt Lake.

The grainy gypsum sand rubbed my skin through my large strap sandals. My open toe stubbed into a small concrete rock. Arms flailed forward as I barely caught my balance, slowing as I recovered.

My father, Randy, tugged at his worn baseball cap with the Air Force Civil Engineering logo embroidered on the front. I heard a muffled laugh before his gruff, flat Midwest accent called to me. "Don't worry about waiting for us, but you may want to keep your balance!"

Planting my feet, I whirled to face my family. Mom's black hair blew across her face, despite the bobby pin tucked behind her ears. Her striped button-down shirt seemed out of place at the lake. She ambled down the slope gingerly, without the abandon of youth or vitality. Dad stood head and shoulders above her, his well-toned arms pushing the handle bars of Dustin's wheelchair. Dustin sat upright, pressing his back hard into his blue foam wheelchair back. He was hesitant to be in a new environment with dangers like water.

I wanted to sprint to the placid lake and be the first to jump in. Instead, I took a deep breath and sighed. I walked back toward my family.

Her cheeks pushed into her eyes as Mom smiled, reaching her arms toward me and tapping her fingers against her palms. She wanted me near. With energy to expend, I sprinted and leaped four feet from her. I landed emphatically at her feet with my heels pushing into the gypsum.

I held Mom's hand, her fingers interlocking with mine, and kicked rocks as I too ambled down the hill. Her hands were slightly chill at the fingers, but soft. I loved her softness. Dad's muscles were hard and rigid, angular and broad. His calf muscles protruded, sculpted by military training. In contrast, Mom's lap was my favorite place to cuddle; her arms felt like a cushion, and her skin was just cool enough, like the underside of a pillow at first cuddle.

At age eleven, I was an inch shorter than Mom. At home I helped her to open jars or close the lock on a window. I walked her pace, Dustin's pace, but my mind barely slowed. I found myself fidgeting, wanting to bolt again towards the water.

Dad, perhaps noticing my physical agitation, took Mom's tender hand with his hairy knuckles and asked me to push Dustin. I moved over and wrapped my fingers around the black protective foam on the handle bar. Dustin's wheelchair was equipped with small thick-rubber grey wheels about twelve inches in diameter. I grunted and strained to push the wide wheels in the sand. It was a sturdy child's wheelchair built more for durability and safety than mobility. Straps hung below the molded foam blue chair. I pushed a strap behind the reinforced metal siding to keep it away from the wheels.

Moving Dustin along at my mother's pace had looked easy with Dad behind the wheels, but I struggled. Leaning my body forward, I dug my heels into the sand and tried to create leverage. I lowered my head and grunted. Pushing was a worthy challenge. Any eleven-year-old could run to the water, but how many of my friends could push this bulky wheelchair with an eight-year-old in it through the sand and not whine? I gritted my teeth and peered down at the deep divots the chair was leaving in the sand and curled my lips into a half smile: I made those marks.

Finally, the wheels caught wet sand; we'd made it to the water. I turned my head toward Dad, who nodded. I loosened my grip on Dustin's wheelchair and unleashed my energy into running like a dog released from the leash. I ran playfully into the water, trying to raise my knees high to gain speed and avoid the resistance against my legs. Being the biggest girl in my fifth grade class, I relished in physical challenge and constantly sought to test my ability. I wanted to be able to lift Dustin and place him gently down rather than awkwardly drop him, push a wheelchair through any type of terrain or incline, and carry my brother as long as, or at least half as long as, Dad could. My increasing strength meant increased family capability. Barely letting my foot pierce the shallow water before quickly picking it up again, I ran thirty yards before the Salt Lake was deep enough to dive into. The splashing salt mixed with the tinge of sweat, matting my hair to my face. Breathing heavily, I placed my palms together with fingers out and leapt into the water, skimming the bottom with my stomach before crawling with my hands. I turned back toward my family and sat waiting.

Standing with water mid-way up his shins, my father had pushed Dustin's wheelchair into the water. My brother sat with his legs crossed in front of his lap, his limber loose muscle allowing his hips double-jointed fluidity. Dustin had both arms behind his neck, keeping all his limbs as far away from the water as possible. Mom languished behind a few paces, standing above the water on a small island of protruding sand. Dad reached into the water and gently splashed some on Dustin's toes, laughing as he did to try to relax Dustin. Dustin recoiled and pushed enough air out to sound like a hiss, bringing his fingers to cover his mouth as he pressed his palm into his cheek. Dad made swirls in the water, splashing every other motion trying to make the water look fun. Dustin timidly let his toe dangle into the water, happily hissed and then he too made swirls in the water.

My lips curled naturally upward; Dustin's joy was so often shared. His closely clipped hair had grown out for a while, giving him a slight cowlick toward the back of his head. His cheeks were chubby and joyful, sagging at the bottom of his jaws. His mouth hung open as his tongue protruded slightly forward past his bottom lip. His eyes were blue and, with his loose muscular facial complexion, usually looked slightly tired. His energy was visible, though, in this new area of sensory perception and adventure; his eyes shined with attentive curiosity as he rippled the water with his toe. He raised his leg, straightened out his knee, and then plunged his whole foot into the water, sending a splash up to his chin. Dustin chortled a genuine, somewhat wheezy, snicker as he enjoyed getting Dad wet with mimicked behavior.

I crawled along the bottom of the Salt Lake as Dustin would often crawl throughout the house since he could not walk, using my elbows to pull along my body as my legs lay behind me, drifting in the water. I pressed my lips together in a child's look of sneaky mischief, submerging my face up to eye level and began to slither towards them as if an alligator after prey. I hummed a poor imitation of the Jaws song under the water and waved my feet to and fro like a tail, trying to be noticed. Dustin saw me and pushed his arms against the bottom of his seat, straightening his back and breathing in with his teeth against his lips. Taking my mouth out of the water, I hummed louder.

"Get her, Dustin! Get her!" Dad bent over to cup water in both hands and threw it at me. Dustin laughed. He tried to kick water at me but didn't get much of a splash with the curve of his foot. He leaned forward with his upper body and moaned, signaling that he wanted in the water.

"Mom! I'm going to need help; they're teaming up on me!" I cried out as Dad unlocked the seat belt like strap buckled across Dustin's waist. The shoulder straps were almost never buckled, except when traveling in vehicles. My parents wanted to give Dustin as much freedom as they could. Tenderly, Dad sat Dustin cross-legged in the water, keeping a hand on Dustin's back for security.

I slithered along the grainy bottom, grinning at Dustin. As Mom approached from behind, I reached out to pinch and wiggle his foot. She grabbed both his shoulders and squeezed, letting out a congested "arrggh." She coughed, stood straight and said, "Little alligator, attack!"

Obediently, I nuzzled my brother's chest, being sure to keep my face out of the water. His chest heaved in excitement. He accepted the cuddling for a second then pushed against me with his forearm.

"I'll give you three seconds to run before I protect my son, little alligator." Dad stuck his oversized hand into the air with three fingers protruding. "Three....two...."

Giggling, I backed up from Dustin and stood up, ready to outrun Dad. I made it five steps. He scooped me off my feet, carried me in both arms for another five steps, then dropped me unceremoniously in the water. I wrestled his leg, trying to make him fall into the water. Dad read me well; he knew when I wanted to test my energy rather than be the dutiful daughter who patiently waited. We played as Dustin and Mom sat placidly where we left them, enjoying the natural scenery and swishing the water about gently to watch the wake.

Later we all joined together to sit in the water. The setting sun blazed across the flat lake, silhouetted by high rising majestic mountains with snow still at the peaks that canvassed across the orange and red hues cast across the Utah sky. Dad pursed his lips together, savoring the transient moment. "Time we head back up the shore," he said.

Dustin's lips were bluish; he was often cold before anyone else. Mom ran her finger across her forehead, tucking her hair behind her ears. We met eyes. She smiled peacefully then ran her finger across my forehead, trying to tame hair ruffled by wind, salt, and sweat.

"Mom, stop. It's not going to do any good anyway." I stood up and offered her my hand. She grabbed my hand with her right and braced by placing her other hand behind her back. I bent my knees for leverage and tried to pull her up. Her lips contorted with the effort.

"I'll just wait for your dad. He'll help me up."

"Yea, after he grabs Dustin..." I let her down and walked towards the wheelchair. Built for a child's safety, the blue wheelchair could carry oxygen tanks. Its wheels had more traction that my mountain bike, and the sides were a flat wall that guarded the inner parts. I wondered if we should have the wheels in salt water. I knew what my parents would say: they didn't want Dustin to miss out on the opportunities of life just to keep his equipment nice. I bent over to move the straps out of the way and readjust the seat for Dustin.

Dad brought Dustin over, his shorts dripping wet and bloated. I didn't want to be the one who had to change that soggy diaper. When Dad placed Dustin in the wheelchair, it was my job to strap him in securely. Dad went over and used two hands to help my mother. I strategically went over to Mom after she had stood up, told her I loved her, and wrapped my arm around her back to walk with her. Dad didn't need the hint; he was already behind the chair.

Tromping back towards the beach, I thought about how we were all together able to adventure at the Great Salt Lake. It wasn't easy to push a wheelchair through water and gypsum. Mom had become more reluctant to physically overexert herself. I was the one who had the most fun. It was mostly for me that we came. Parents in Utah seem to be required to let their children swim in the Great Salt Lake at least once, however unpleasant the water smelled. My parents wanted me to have that. I stared wistfully at the mountains across the vista. I imagined running alone with a backpack down a trail, jumping from rock to rock and leaping over streams. I'd never be able to do that with my family.

"Thanks for bringing us here, Dad. I enjoyed it."

His face brightened. "The best part is still to come. I have a blanket and sandwiches in the car for our picnic."

I took a picture of them that day. It's one of my favorite memories.

***

The childhood toy bought most often for my brother was a helium balloon. Dustin loved the chaotic movement of a balloon when hit and the predictable return of a balloon when tethered to a weight. Around age ten, my brother became much more mobile as his muscles continued to grow stronger, and he could operate his wheelchair proficiently on his own. Every shopping trip, Dustin's wheelchair would be pushed by Dad, Mom, or me, and as soon as

Dustin recognized where the balloons were, he would wheel himself in the general direction of the balloons visible along the ceiling line. His body had developed better than expected, and at that point he was able to feed himself, breathe without assistance, sleep without the BiPAP machine, and maneuver around the house.

By age ten, Dustin could push his wheelchair towards the balloons at a faster pace than I walked. He would roll under the balloons, looking for a Mickey Mouse or Barney balloon, unless there was a particularly shiny one to lure him. Dustin still couldn't walk on his own, although the public education system did help him learn to walk next to rails for a few steps and increase the amount of time he could stand next to something. Due to a lack of body control and his adventurous impulses, Dustin would be strapped in across his waist whenever we traveled with his wheelchair. After picking his balloon, my brother would point and motion and give a grunt from deep in his stomach to ask me to grab the one he wanted.

I would pull the chord of the balloon I thought Dustin wanted, present it to him, and see if he agreed with my choice. Dustin's sign for joy from his wheelchair was to straighten his legs, lock his knees, hunch his shoulders, bring his hands to his face, and hiss with a heavy outward breath of excitement. If I picked the right balloon, that was his response. If I picked the wrong balloon, he would point and grunt at another. On his ambitious days, he would grab the balloon with his left hand and point at another with his right hand.

Dustin loved to smack a balloon and watch it jump out and return to his wheelchair where it was tethered. He enjoyed hitting the edge of the balloon to make it spin in place. He relished in chaotic hits that resulted in spin and velocity. However, Dustin's favorite part was the shiny silver backing where he could stare at his reflection. Dustin enjoyed the unpredictable results of a heavy swing, but his greatest fascination was with light and refraction.

Flashlights allured my brother. He would giggle incessantly while holding a flashlight next to his cheek under his eyeball. Sometimes he would even stick the flashlight right in front of his eye, staring straight into the light. My parents would stop him from using a flashlight in that particular way when they caught him. He also liked to trace the light along the ceiling, using his flexibility from loose muscles to sit comfortably with his head lounging backward so that the back of his head almost touched his back, giggling and hissing as he moved the light. If I were playing with him, I would make the light dance, jumping it around from spot to spot on the floor, to the wall, on his leg, etc. Like a cat, he enjoyed trying to chase the light and sometimes jolted when it moved.

Dustin enjoyed life's simple grandeurs. From grade school until high school I would come home, help my mother get Dustin off the bus, get him changed and situated, do my homework, then play games like these with my brother. As a mother, I again appreciate these types of moments with Eli playing humble games. However, raising Eli has also brought new eyes of revelation to Dustin's unique condition. At eighteen months old, my son could complete knob puzzles, connect magnetic toy trains in a series, sit and pretend to read his own book, walk, run, and jump off the couch. In physical and vocal ability, Eli outpaced Dustin by the time Eli was about eleven months old. Sweeping the floor and attempting to fold his own clothes are things my brother never attempted. I asked my son if he needed a diaper change and he ran away saying 'no' and tried to hide in the closet, in between his father's legs. Dustin never developed the motivation to hide, deceive, or mislead. In many ways, he stayed innocent.

Dustin's life wasn't about accomplishments. He didn't judge by abilities. People were worthwhile to him because they smiled at him, not because of what they could do. While life was hard for Dustin, his joys were simple and therefore many. Dustin was happy without expensive toys or the newest device. He didn't need brand name clothes. Dustin embodied the joy of human interaction without the worry of ownership or achievement.

My needs weren't as simple. I accumulated a sizable collection of computer game CDs. He got the first one by accident. When I left one of my favorite games on the edge of the computer desk, my brother scooted over and grabbed the CD. He was first drawn to his own reflection on the backside of the disk. Then he began to rotate his wrist, bringing out the iridescent colors. I found the scratched disk later with a raspberry of slobber on the backside. I imagine he used the same expression of joy as when receiving a balloon – bringing his hands and the CD to his mouth and letting out an excited breath of hiss and slobber. Needless to say, my CD was ruined, but Dustin had discovered a new toy. After that, my family regularly supplied him with bygone games and old Windows operating systems.

So much of what we value in life is temporary, a new fad interposing itself between deeper meaning and our focus. Dustin would destroy more than one of my valued CDs. It wasn't often that I yelled at my brother, but in my immaturity I often blamed my parents and fussed at them for not taking better care of their son.

It was near impossible to take care of Dustin, keep a spotless house, and make sure none of my 'valuables' were destroyed. When I was young it was hard to see past my own needs. Knowing the undercurrents of how Mom's adult onset myotonic dystrophy was affecting her as I grew older, perhaps my largest regret from my teenage years is my lack of patience I had with my parents. The value of life isn't in how well we control the objects we think we own, but it's hard to keep focused on what matters.

Chapter 4
September 23

Pondering my future as a junior in high school, I began to marvel at my luck at birth. Myotonic dystrophy led me to question my blessings. From our mother, Dustin inherited a disease which necessitated a wheelchair. I had the genetics that created a muscle structure able to pursue school records in the weight room. Why could I sprint down a basketball court while my brother sat in his wheelchair? Should I be allowed to dream of being a college athlete when it had been said of Dustin that he would die before he graduated high school? Why had I won writing contests, excelled in school, and had an individual education plan in school because of a high IQ? My brother lacked the ability to form sentences. In school he never wrote. His individual education plan included learning how to separate and shred paper and repetitively push the same button on command. Why was I was born capable?

Doctors said I didn't seem to have inherited myotonic dystrophy, but I still didn't understand why I had so many natural advantages and Dustin had so many unfortunate disabilities. Luck was a poor explanation. I searched for answers, even in X-Men comic books, trying to find a reason I was given health.

Were my gifts given in visible contrast to my brother's so I would know how fortunate I was? Three years older than my brother, I grew up doing adult caretaking tasks. Through the years, I would change thousands of diapers, brush Dustin's teeth, lift him into bed, administer nebulizer treatments, clean his feeding tube, watch him when both my parents had to work, bathe him, unload his wheelchair from the bus, and play with him. I didn't always think I was fortunate.

Was I healthy so I could grow up to help others like my brother? I dreamed of working with children like Dustin after I graduated college. I imagined the joy on faces like Dustin's as I played puppets for a living. I thought I could love that work because I had been raised to give acts of love in taking care and playing with those whom society might otherwise leave behind.

While I survived most of my brother's life with a blind optimism, throwing quarters in wishing wells and praying to an unseen God, not questioning why my life was the way it was, when I was sixteen my idyllic childhood clashed against the hard reality of what a terminal disease meant.

***

I woke up September 23, 2002, to the sound of a 6:30 a.m. alarm. I rolled over in bed, squinted with my weak vision to see the clock, sighed, stretched a body sore in the hips, shoulders, and thighs from wall jumps at volleyball practice and slowly rolled out of bed. I turned off the alarm and opened the drawers to dress for school. I packed my practice shoes, hair band, and books, gathered my homework from the previous night, and slung my backpack across my shoulders.

I walked up stairs, dropped my backpack by the door, and went to heat up some oatmeal for breakfast. Dustin was napping on the living room floor. Dustin had a cold, a common enough occurrence after surviving thirteen years with myotonic dystrophy and a weak immune system. As flexible as he was with his loose muscles, his favorite way to sleep was to have his legs in front of him with toes turned slightly inward and knees resting comfortably touching the floor while his chest rested in between his legs on the ground and his head turned off to the side.

By age thirteen, Dustin was rather large, his body beginning to show effects of puberty. He had more hair on his face, including eyebrows that almost touched in the middle and thin black hairs on his upper lip. His right eye had begun to drift from astigmatism. If he were a normal thirteen-year-old, the same dentist who had recommended I get braces probably would have recommended Dustin get braces so that he could have a straight set of teeth into adulthood.

His frame was slender, with grasshopper-like legs that had never seen the muscle building exercise of walking a city block. His arms were more substantial from throwing his wheels forward in his wheelchair, revealing how much stronger his muscles had become since having open heart surgery and the days of eating through a tube. His rotund belly protruded more than it would have if his abdominal muscles had more strength. He loved to share Dad's Mountain Dew and Cheetos. In the year prior, Dustin had probably grown about three inches and stood past the shoulders of my five foot ten frame. Dad could still handle Dustin's weight easily, but Dustin had grown past Mom's carrying capacity. Getting Dustin in and out of bed when Dad was gone had become my responsibility. Along with the hair on his upper lip, puberty had brought Dustin's weight to over ninety pounds. He seemed to be on track to become six feet tall like the other Bartz boys in the family. Lifting him was like hoisting a bushel of corn with sacks of potatoes for appendages.

Dustin's cold meant I didn't have to help Mom dress, feed, or load Dustin into his wheelchair to get ready for school. I had an extra twenty minutes in my morning routine. I went back down stairs to check social media. After wasting enough time, I came upstairs, rested my hand on the doorknob, and stopped to watch Dustin before I headed to school. He lay in an awkward position, head resting comfortably forward between his two legs. His secondhand red shirt was bigger than necessary, and his sleeping sweats were worn and too short. The curve of his calf muscle was submerged in the folds of his shirt as his chest rested on the ground between his knees. I stared at his back, watching for breath.

He hadn't made much noise at all that morning, no joyful laughs or excited grunts. He lay there quietly like an overused Stretch Armstrong doll. It was a rare morning when I had time in the morning to log into a computer. He had gotten sick Thursday night and not recovered enough to go to school Monday. It had been awhile since he missed two consecutive days of school.

I'd always measured my brother's years against the doctor's estimates of his life span. He had already bypassed so many 'clocks' set on his fragile body. I watched and waited, taking a few breaths myself while waiting on Dustin's first. I lingered at the door, something inside of me wanting to go hug or hold him, and something else saying it was just another day. I needed to head to school. Finally, his chest heaved up with the center of his back moving slowly as his ribs expanded outward heavily towards the capacity of his breath and descended down in a quicker motion. I can still see that eternal blink of a moment when I close my eyes.

In class that morning, I sat in metal chair with a hard blue plastic base. I had a high B in a chemistry class with the reputation of having more students with Fs than As. I had studied for a test about molecular mass in bonded compounds and sat trying to solve the given equation, drawing some symbol like CL for chlorine and placing dots around to represent the electrons. The phone rang. Mrs. Moore, her chin length dark brown hair in tight small curls, answered in her business voice. Students didn't make random noises in her class to interrupt tests; neither should the phone. I finished my calculation and tried to reread the question to double check my answer. The phone interruption broke my concentration. I looked up at her stern face with a few age lines and trim athletic figure as she said, "Yes, she is, but she is taking a test." The unheard reply from the other end elicited an unexpected response: "Oh, I see. I'll send her right down." Her eyes locked with mine. Usually, her eyes were somewhat narrow, peering out with obvious intelligence and a task-oriented personality from behind thick glasses. When she looked at me her eyes were wide, her usually calm demeanor unsettled.

"Darcy, come to my desk. Bring your test." I walked to her desk, feeling a dread somewhere between test anxiety and the foreboding that lingered always at the back of my mind when Dustin was not in my range of vision. My footsteps reverberated; a silent classroom's attention shifted from the test and fell upon my back. Mrs. Moore smiled at me, the practiced smile of the woman who had served as a local city commissioner. During a difficult test in an academically competitive class, this smile did not succeed in reassuring me. She had always been polite and responsive, but I had never seen her purposefully try to be warm toward me before. My nerves were on edge.

Her voice still held its command of authority, yet something gentle snuck out. "There is someone to speak to you in the office. Please head there right away." I put my test on her desk, asking a question with my eyes to see if that were acceptable, not daring to speak during her test. She nodded, blinked, and returned to grading the test stack already on her desk. I walked toward the classroom door. Thoughts of chlorine or electrons evaporated. What in the world could happen to get me called out of Mrs. Moore's test?

I opened the classroom door, carefully closed it behind me, and took two steps in the hallway. I heard my own voice, or a voice, or my own thought on a different brain wave length – whatever it was: "Darcy, your brother is dead." My skin went cold. My fingers tingled. My shoe stopped moving on the tile. I shook my head, closed my eyes, and relived the way his chest rose and fell as I stood at the door that morning. He breathed. I took a long drink at the water fountain. Dustin had survived too much for a cold to cause this much nervous energy. I cleared my mind, girding for the rest of the walk to the office.

The water fountain was at the edge of the wall, opening to a central area by a main entrance where a wooden carving of the school mascot Mustang sat on a pedestal. I'd climbed the stairs to my left every school day that year. It was a Monday about eight weeks into my third school year in the building. I was where I was supposed to be; I'd walked this hallway a thousand times before. I took a deep breath, put my eyes on the floor just in front of my feet, and followed the pattern of maroon and white square tiles to the office.

When I entered the office, the secretary wore an overly kind smile, with eyes looking at me as Mrs. Moore's did after the phone call. I opened my mouth, but the secretary pointed to my parents, who were standing in the middle of the open area in the office. Dad stood with his arm wrapped around Mom's shoulder, her eyes puffy, downcast. Her shoulders sagged as she leaned on Dad. She looked at him. He nodded, turned towards me, and gave a weak smile. His voice was gruff, like used sandpaper to be worn down again: "Darcy, your mother has something to tell you."

Mom remained still. Her hair was in a loose black ponytail, stray gray hairs escaping near her bangs. She leaned against Dad, who bore the brunt of her weight. Exhaustion exuded from her. She lifted her tired face. Her bloodshot blue eyes met mine. She was different -- older, sad.

Perhaps the last breath I watched my brother take gave it away. Maybe it was my mother's eyes. I knew what she wanted to say.

Her hand closed in a fist against Dad's chest, her posture so slack that her shoulders were barely visible. Her mouth opened, then closed again, and I thought of how much Dustin's chin resembled Mom's. Spittle stuck to the corners of her lips, and her tear ducts welled. Her tremulous voice pushed out the words. "Your brother passed away this morning."

These moments in life are surreal: intangibly fast, yet timeless. I kept a dream journal at that age in hopes of self-discovery. The two weeks prior were littered with entries, perhaps premonitions, about death – odd dreams more symbolic than understandable. Maybe I read more into those entries looking back than I recognized going forward, but something in my life understood what was coming. I heard my mother's words, but I don't remember thinking or deciding anything. The oddly friendly smiles, the voice in the hallway, my parent's body language, Dustin's chest heaving slow and heavy: my mother told me my brother was dead, and I said, "I know."

I did know. Perhaps it was logical, my subconscious mind putting together the clues that look so obvious in retrospect, like a well-plotted mystery novel. Perhaps it was a sibling connection, or perhaps it was just time that the doctor's guesses were right. I had expected my brother's death for years. I stood there looking at my parents, living the reality I had accepted and, in some senses, prepared for, since I was three years old.

"I knew you'd know," Mom said in a stabilizing, more confident, yet still husky voice. A smile broke across her face in the relief of her only remaining child not being shocked by the death of her youngest. She smiled genuinely, perhaps for the first time since cradling Dustin's body as the fire truck alarm blared towards the house in response to her 911 call. Her son had died that morning in her arms as she tried resuscitating him with her own breath, but the first indication of her daughter's reaction was calm. The child raised to expect death met the first moments of the news with seeming serenity.

I remember standing there, just standing. It's like looking back at a photograph that was never taken – time stood still. It's as if a black hole existed in that moment as I swam through the depths of fear meeting faith, the inevitable and the known crashing up against the new unknown territory. As much as I've thought about that day, those moments of shock are elusive, tendrils of a time where my body froze and my whole world shifted. I stood there while my parents hugged, not knowing what to do with myself, not knowing how to feel, not knowing what to think.

Principal Stett invited us into his office to have a private place to sit and talk. We walked past the secretary's desk full of Post It notes and stacks of paper through a doorway to a small room with a circle table and four chairs. He politely closed the door behind us. I heard the soft scruff of plastic on carpet as he pulled out my chair. The walls were clean and white with a soft scent of lavender, a conference room for calming students. As soon as I sat, I wailed – deep, hollow potent tears. I cried from my lungs, my stomach, the back of my throat, the bottom of my spine, through my mouth, and through my nose. The noises came before the tears, but tears spurted quickly and surged down my cheeks. Immediately I felt the pain in my throat. Guttural gasps of air escaped through my constricted larynx. The white walls and closed doors ramified the sound. All I heard was my own weeping. My nostrils flared, and snot trickled to the tip of my lip. My hands shook until I clenched my hands into fists, slumped my head on my arm, and vented the hot breath of anguish onto the table.

Everyone in the office heard me, my heart laid bare, the calm serenity of knowing obliterated in the sudden cataclysm of living without Dustin.

I had stood and watched him breathe; he should have been safe. I should have been able to come home to hug him and say I loved him. I watched him breathe and left. I stopped to watch him breathe because I knew something wasn't right, and then I left. I couldn't go back to the moment. I left.

He was gone, and I was left. The race against the ticking time clock of his terminal disease was gone, and the pain was left. The hope was gone, and the anger was left. My prior way of life was gone, but I was left.

Chapter 5
Noah's Ark and Walks to the Park

Life with Dustin had been ruled by necessary routine, with certain time-consuming caretaker tasks that had to be done every day. Each weekday in the morning Mom would get Dustin out of bed, change his diaper, dress him for the day, pack his bag, brush his teeth, and meet the school bus in the driveway. When Dustin got home, we would change his diaper and his clothes if he drooled too much that day, take off his foot splints and shoes, relax with him a while before bath, bathe him, dress him for bed, brush his teeth, put him in bed, and put the guard rail up. There was no off day in taking care of Dustin. For years, Mom, Dad and I all lived with a daily routine of caring for someone with greater than normal needs. It was stabilizing, comforting, and an act of love to give such care. After September 23, 2002, those routines were gone.

I was the daughter of a career military man. Routine was how we survived. I clung to routine wherever I could still find it. I returned to school as quickly as possible. On the night of Dustin's viewing I played in a volleyball game, hoping to feel normal, to be able to move on with my goals without letting my world fall into the chaos. My family, which had come to the funeral home in Nebraska Cornhusker red, entered the gym as a horde adorned in the same way. I needed an escape, a way to force the thoughts in my head to silence. The routine of a volleyball game was my answer.

Tying my laces in the locker room, I willed my fingers to work, consciously battled my body to be goal-driven rather than lethargic. I sat down on the bench with my shoes on, laid my head in my hands, took slow deep breaths, and willed down the impulse to lie down and cry myself to sleep. During warm-ups, I ran focused on the sounds of sneakers hitting the gym floor reverberating, trying to numb my active thoughts. The acrid taste of adrenaline meeting exhaustion swirled in my mouth, and I swallowed it down, happy to have something I knew how to battle.

I wanted an escape. My focused willpower funneled on that volleyball court. Routine meant a distraction from the inevitable upheaval ahead.

It was a different level of athletic focus, a form of escape in which my whole existence centered on that court or crumbled. Tingling with competitive spirit, I stared and smiled at the girl I planned to serve to next. I was audaciously competitive, enlivened by the adrenaline in a body that had gone stoic from shock. I played without restraint or complicity, seeking an acceptable yet primal way to feel something besides a passive hope and blind optimism in God's plan that didn't seem so easy any more. During that game, I was alive. During that game, I forgot my brother was dead.

I didn't feel emotion during the game; I felt adrenaline. After the game, I walked back from the locker room into a gym empty except my family, dressed in Nebraska red. I remembered the funeral home, faced reality again. Exhaustion set in, my legs weighed down like a horse sinking into quicksand. My sweat dried into a clammy film, cold across my forehead. I didn't want to leave, to go face the task of writing a eulogy for my brother. That gym was a temporary sanctuary, a reprieve to reality. I wanted that moment to last, to pretend the glories of high school JV volleyball could save me from my only brother's death.

I hugged my family, made the necessary small talk, went home to my writing table, and wrote. At age sixteen I read this at Dustin's funeral on the September 26:

> I've spent many a day just looking at my brother and wondering what it was I saw. He would stare at me with a child's innocence, laugh at a random something, and burst into spontaneous action. You never could anticipate that little guy. He played life by a different set of rules.
>
> His perspective was unique, his conscious built on a different level of thought. It's said that when you lack in one sense, you make it up in others, and while my

brother may not have been gifted with the ability of words, he had a direct way of speaking to the heart. You looked in his eyes and saw him laugh, a laugh containing an innocent purity. You'd hold his hand to comfort him, and feel comforted by him.

They say life is tough, a 'school of hard knocks,' but from Dustin I learned life to be candid and filled with simple joys. He wasn't burdened by other's thoughts of him, or money, or obligation. He lived a life as given to him by God. He lived as the closest thing I've seen to a pure soul. He wasn't burdened by the material world; instead he embraced it, bent his reality to his own joys, and bent our perspective by living his life.

You may think it was hard to grow up Dustin's sister. Perhaps it did have restrictions of sorts, giving me a different life. However, I would disagree, as this life is all I've known, and my character in a large part is formed by being blessed with the opportunity to live and experience with Dustin. I know I am what I am today because the lessons Dustin brought to me. My perspective on the world has Dustin's influence as a corner stone. I catch myself laughing at nothing, finding joy from the oddest things. Sometimes I wake up with a sense of naïve wonder, innocent curiosity. There's so much of my life, and the value in it, that I owe to my brother. I thank God that Dustin was able to touch my life being just the way he was.

My brother is a part of my character, and I will strive all of my life to hold to the virtues and values I learned with him as a part of my life. I'm glad he was with us. May he make the angels as happy.

I'd like to share a poem about my brother:

Dustin Ryan Bartz

Noah's Ark and walks to the park
Ice cream saloon and hot air balloon,
Licky-licky and puppets of Mickey
Yucky slobber and a loving clobber
Key taker and noise maker
Innocent child, boy gone wild
Morning cartoon, always a loon
Never a fuss for the school bus
Pet a mutt and wiggle your butt
Splashing in the bath, where lead his path?
Always a fighter, now with a burden lighter
Little boy, big joy
He wasn't here long but sang a touching song
Lived a different way, showed love every day
Dustin Ryan Bartz… touched many hearts.

After I delivered that poem and walked down the steps to my seat, I collapsed into Mom's arms and wailed. My friends all saw me cry, many for the first time, some not for the last.

For someone who never said a full sentence, Dustin had a wide and positive impact on the people who crossed his path. I admired Dustin, loved him, even envied his innocence. I struggled with the way the world was after Dustin's death more. I had been raised all my life to expect my brother to die before me, to believe that was God's plan, and to cherish each day with my brother in the meantime. As a child, I felt blessed, as if I were given a window into heaven by living with someone connected to the heart of God's plan, graced each day with an Angel's blessing of love and good cheer. As a child, I thought myotonic dystrophy was one of God's unique gifts given to special children to be blessings on earth.

Living in a family with a terminally ill child is like that. Your hope and outlook are tested daily by such extreme odds that you build up a fervent hope, a blind optimism, perhaps even a calloused denial of what reality offers. Some children grow up believing in Santa, the Tooth fairy, or that they can 'be anything' they want to be. My family raised me without a belief in Santa or the tooth fairy. Dad helped me understand probability and natural limits when I told him I wanted to be the first female player in Major League Baseball. While I read fantasy books and played video games, I had a good sense was what was and what wasn't. I was raised fairly grounded in reality. Except perhaps with my brother.

As a child, I poured myself into goals of helping Dustin learn to talk, or sign, or walk. I prayed every day that my brother would become healthier and stronger and live longer. Dustin defied the odds for so long that my young mind believed miracles happened often. I prayed fervently for the miracle of a cure every night. That is one of the greatest gifts I received in being Dustin's sister. I learned to pray, wanting what I prayed for with all of my heart, with an unquestioned simplicity and an innate trust that my prayers mattered. I believed those prayers were part of why Dustin did so well. Perhaps they were.

I haven't been able to pray with the same unquestioned simplicity of hope since Dustin passed. My childhood ended the day my brother died. The naive hope that a miracle would save him, that he would one day walk, that a disease was a blessing in my family – that hope died with him.

Chapter 6
As the Sirens Became Audible

Mom didn't talk much about the day Dustin died. Dad told me the basics. Most of what Mom did tell me, she didn't reveal until years later. Here is the story of that morning.

His last morning, Dustin lay with his head between his legs, doubled over and sleeping in a position etched in my brain from the morning I stood to watch him breathe and left. Mom didn't get to leave and focus on something else like I did; she worked around the house and waited for him to wake. She monitored his breathing. She witnessed the intervals between breaths become longer, waited for another breath.

She watched. His back rose, slowly arching, expanding feebly, reaching a premature crest. His back fell, empty, exhausted. Her eyes stayed fixed on his back. It didn't move. Each second of waiting, she inched closer, wondering if her eyes deceived her, if she just needed to be nearer to see the movement. Finally, she stood over him, next to him, and still didn't see breath. She leaned in, placed her finger tips on his back – no movement. She pressed down, and his back fell more. Empty. Exhausted.

Panic swelled in her chest. Both her hands joined together to shake his back, trying to jostle him from sleep. A yelp of air escaped – from her own throat. "Dustin!"

Frantically, she pushed him from his sitting slumber, laying him on his back. She laid a palm forcefully on his chest and, with her right hand on top, attempted to force air into his lungs with compressions. One, two, three. His chest seemed to rise again – was it breath?

She swabbed his mouth with her finger, looking for a clog, trying to free the airways. Nothing but cold spittle. She tiled his chin back, lifting her fingers beneath his skin. The tears on her cheek felt warmer than her son.

She wailed in pain, fear emanated from her. His lips were a shade too blue. Her fingers pinched his nose, his head tilted back. Lip to lip, she tried to once again give her son life. Her breath entered his lungs. Did his come out? She never said.

She dashed for the phone, dialed 911, and tried to cry clearly enough for the respondent to understand.

She returned to him, tried again and again and again. She held him cradled in her arms as the sirens became audible. She prayed it wasn't good-bye; she knew it was beyond her power. "Lord, give me one more day. Give me one more day with my son."

She nestled her nose into his neck, a neck without pulse, a neck without motion. The firefighter rushed through the door. Did he speak to her? How many men came in? What did she do next? Mom never said.

Dustin was pronounced dead on arrival.

Mom was the only one home. She was the one traumatized by hearing the fire truck sirens while holding her dying, perhaps dead, son. She was the one who gave him CPR to try to save him. She held him during and after his last breaths. She fought to give him his last breaths. She passed on the genetic code that brought about his last breaths so soon. She couldn't prolong that life any longer. His time came because of a disease inherited from her genetics. She was powerless to stop it.

The guilt never left her. I remember when she first pointed to the spot where Dustin had been lying when she realized his breaths were gone. Her eyes were distant, her voice hollow. Mom had changed.

Chapter 7
Parenting Through the Pain

My parents both worked the graveyard shift together at Wal-Mart after Dustin passed away. The extra dollar per hour mattered, but working together meant neither felt as alone at work. Even then Dad was trying to care for Mom. He had been groomed in the role of caretaker for thirteen years. The heart habit of sacrificing for his family didn't end with Dustin's death.

Being home alone wasn't fun for any of us after Dustin took his last breath in the corner of the living room near the stairs. Mom worked at the dressing room, and Dad stocked shelves. I'd visit Wal-Mart to buy essentials, browse clothes I'd never buy, or simply to find Mom and know my family was still near. She always wore my softball button with a picture of my smiling face with windblown hair. It wasn't the most flattering picture, but Mom never left for work without it.

When I went in to Wal-Mart late at night, Mom would want to show me off to her co-workers. She would smile and brag about whatever it was she could in my recent athletic or academic career. It was embarrassing, but I was glad for the company and happy to get away from a quiet house at night.

Working as a dressing room attendant was her happiest position at Wal-Mart. There she could sit in a chair when needed, answer the phone, and help restock the shelves. Her job was within her physical ability, gave her a social circle of coworkers, and let her interact and be seen in the community. She had become a dressing room attendant only after a few years of cashiering, a job that became increasingly difficult for her. She found it hard to make her scanning quotas and standing for hours hurt her legs. She had requested to move to the dressing room to spend less time on her feet.

For many years, since 1996, Mom worked in retail stores. In Utah she worked three years at Target, and in Kansas she had worked almost seven years at Wal-Mart. Perhaps working to long in one spot led to boredom. Maybe her coworkers talked to her less. Maybe there was a conflict. Whatever it was, Mom requested a position change away from being a dressing room attendant. She put in for the bakery and didn't get it, was turned down to be a door greeter, and couldn't work with Dad in loading due to her inability to carry heavy weights. Management offered her a cashier job again, which she accepted.

If cashiering was hard on her body before, it was even harder this time. She wasn't able to stand long, so she requested to be able to sit in a chair like she could at the dressing rooms. Cashiers don't sit in chairs often at Wal-Mart. She was told no. She requested to go back to the dressing room but the position was filled. She tried to do her duty as a cashier but was slow, felt pain in her legs, didn't meet quotas, and felt like she wasn't living up to expectations. She needed a chair, and for that she was told she needed a doctor's note from a company-approved doctor. The doctor she went to told her that her disease did not affect women and that her symptoms were not from MMD but her depression. He had never treated another patient with MMD, which has clear empirical evidence and many examples of affecting women. He must have confused it with another variant of muscular dystrophy. He didn't write her a note to get a chair.

After more discussions with her boss, Mom finally was reassigned to the cigarette aisle cashier, where she would be allowed to use a chair. She felt pressure to be able to scan a certain number of items per hour. The cigarette aisle didn't get as much traffic. She wished she was more capable at a job that she had excelled at seven years ago. She wanted to be able to stand longer without pain like she was once able to. Her inability to do what she once did well began to damage her self-worth.

From the outside, it may have seemed my mother needed to 'toughen up' and learn to adapt to the changes in her older body – something everyone experiences. However, degenerative muscular diseases take a hidden toll. Studies have estimated over half of families with an adult suffering from myotonic dystrophy also experience poverty.

As the disease worsened, Mom was less capable of working long hours and experienced muscle fatigue earlier in an eight hour shift. Her body became less capable of standing. Her sleep patterns suffered due to lack of oxygen. Poor oxygenation during sleep can cause mental fatigue and slower mental reactions. The combination of poor sleep oxygenation, excessive daytime sleepiness, and increasing muscle pain and weakness made daily routines more difficult. Drooping facial muscles affected her appearance. Remembering where she put something took more effort. Abstract concepts were harder to understand verbally. Mom began to feel less useful, have less confidence, and feel guilty about her capabilities. A good and diligent worker, she was once and wanted to continue to be a quality employee. Her body wasn't as capable as before. In my naïve high school attitude, I tried to motivate her to be tougher mentally, to push through it. Mom's trouble with work coincided with her grief after Dustin's passing, and maybe that was why it was hard to see what her adult onset MMD was doing to her body.

Many mothers sacrifice career advancement for their children, but this is especially true for mothers of children with life threatening disease. My parents made many sacrifices in their ability to gain new skills or to progress in a given career field to care for Dustin. Mom had a two year degree from New Mexico State University in Alamogordo. Yet she sacrificed her time to develop a career so Dustin felt loved, even when hooked to hospital machines.

Mom worked restaurant jobs, was a para-educator in the school systems, tried selling Avon products from home, and worked in retail during opposite hours of Dad so that Dustin could be cared for by those who knew his needs best and loved him genuinely. She put her children first. However, when Dustin passed away, Mom was often the only one home. She'd cry alone in the living room. She visibly cringed at the sound of fire engines. Her role as caretaker for her son ended in traumatizing moments that left a scar on her psyche.

She held her son in her arms as he took his dying breaths and could not save him. Mom's diminishing skills were not the lone factor in her declining ability to hold a job. Many adult parents suffering from MMD also have to bear the death of a child. An adult with MMD might have a child with more severe symptoms. A mother might hold her child in his last breaths as she knows the disease she gave him robs his heart of the ability to beat longer. A woman with adult onset MMD might have to experience depression, battle through the death of a child, cope with her own degeneration, and fight the unknown effects of the disease on her breathing ability, her sleep patterns, and the oxygenation to her brain.

My mother did.

Living with Mom, I did not always feel the empathy and compassion toward her that I now do. As a typical child of a normal-looking woman, I thought Mom should be more like I pictured myself to be, more like she seemed in the memories. As a high school student contemplating college, I worried about my own economic future. I felt anger and resentment at my parents, as they had trouble feeling satisfied from working a low wage, forty hour a week job after Dustin passed away. I saved every dollar I could for college and wanted my parents to hold steady jobs too much to empathize with the difficulty. I thought I needed Mom to keep working a job that made her feel worthless and weak. If she quit, my future might be limited, my ability to fit in or find success harder. In my mind, she needed to find a way to move beyond Dustin's death and actively search for some coping mechanism outside of work. That way at work she could focus, feel happy, and perform her duties without her sadness getting in the way. My naive viewpoint added to her depression. I didn't get it.

Looking at the numbers, the signs, the symptoms, it makes sense that a woman with MMD who had a son with MMD would have a family flirting with the poverty line. We would have been well below the poverty line if not for my father's twenty year military career and retirement pay. Dad's dutiful military service saved us from the tragic economic patterns which can be common to families with degenerative genetic disease. Even then, the only year I was not on free lunch during high school was the year after Dustin passed away.

We had one less dependent and the paperwork didn't account for the funeral bills on a child life insurance companies didn't want to cover.

After retiring from the military and then losing his son, Dad cycled through many jobs in a short span of time. Eventually, Dad ended up driving two hours away to Larned, Kansas, on Mondays. He would sleep at his brother's, Michael's, house, then work a three or four day work week with lots of overtime with Bartz Plumbing, Heating, and Cooling. Unlike many of the entry level positions Dad had shifted through, this job utilized Dad's skills he developed in the military. He was happy working with his brother. He felt skilled, well paid, and had the humanizing effect of working for a boss who knew what had transpired recently in his life.

Mom had quit working by then and could often be found home alone. Traveling to my college softball games was one of my parents' biggest priorities; however, it happened less with Dad commuting two hours for work. Mom began to feel lonely, and Dad felt travel-worn. During my senior year of college my parents decided to move to Larned so Dad could work full-time with his brother. The job paid commensurate with his skill and benefited his family. Mom left the home Dustin died in to see her husband more.

My parents had talked often about moving. Dad had a nomadic spirit after twenty years in the military. At one point, they had wanted to move back to Mom's home town of Alamogordo, New Mexico. However, the economic outlook would not have been as beneficial. Dad, although skilled, did not pursue a college degree and instead entered the military after high school. While twenty years of service to one's country builds a great deal of character and capability, writing a resume or cover letter wasn't something he did often in the Air Force.

In Larned, Dad had a job where his boss recognized and appreciated his skills and physical strength, knew his background, and valued him as a person. His last job in the Air Force had been as a plant operator at the base's water treatment plant. He was a respected leader in charge of enlisted and civilian workers. Such a work environment was hard to recreate as a forty-five-year-old-plus worker with no college experience and the type of transient life that made it hard to track addresses for references and letters of recommendation. Working for Bartz Plumbing, Heating, and Cooling was ideal. His work made him feel accomplished, his physical strength came in handy, and he cared to perform well for his boss. Working for his brother in labor worth doing helped Dad move on from Dustin's death and find himself again in the sweat and grime of a job he enjoyed.

Mom's work experience in the small western Kansas town of Larned was not so fortunate. Larned had a shrinking population of just over 4,000. At first, Mom didn't desire work. Between Dad's military retirement, his twice monthly paychecks, and the lack of dependent children, he could support himself and his wife. They rented for a time, saved enough money, and bought a house. They invested in a new Ford Focus to drive to see my senior year of softball and help my mother feel more comfortable on car trips as travel became harder on her body. Financially, they could meet their monthly needs, travel, and save for an annual trip to visit Mom's family.

Money to survive wasn't the reason Mom wanted to work again. Living in a small town with few connections, she felt like an outsider. She would go on weekly trips to the library to play Mahjong tiles or Phase 10, but once I graduated from college and no longer had softball games, Mom wasn't a regular part of a social group she enjoyed. The military life takes its toll on wives, and Mom had moved around and sacrificed so many hours for her children that she didn't have many long-term relationships outside of family. While she enjoyed spending time with Dad's brother, Michael, his wife Sandi, and their three children, she didn't find the same community heartfelt warm embrace Dad found. In Larned, Mom had no one genetically similar to her, a hard situation for a woman with a rare disease.

Michael's boys played sports year round and rode horses or four-wheelers on their open country property. Mom didn't have the physical capability or interest for athletics, a central social activity in small-town Kansas. Dad would go to many Bartz boys' sporting events, from recreation league baseball to middle school football to high school basketball games. He fit in the small country community atmosphere. Unfortunately, Mom rarely felt that same rapport.

Mom may not have been a social butterfly in Salina, but she was known in a positive way, and many people enjoyed talking with her. People in Salina remembered her deceased son, and cared about her active daughter. The only people in Larned who would have known Dustin would have been family. While family helps, she missed people understanding part of what she went through. When my parents visited Salina after moving to Larned, they would find a reason to go shop at Wal-Mart and spend more time chatting with former co-workers than shopping. Working helped Mom meet some of her social needs and connected her with a group of people who cared. Humans are social creatures. Mom was no exception.

Mom lost her way of life when she lost Dustin. She lost the good-willed communication that people give a mother of a child in a wheelchair. She would still talk to the parents at my sporting events after Dustin passed away, but sitting in those same stands sometimes reminded her more of what she lost than the game playing out in front of her. Mom would still host people at the house, but being in that recliner next to where he took his last breaths had to remind her more of who wasn't in the room than who was. Any mother who loses a child is changed.

When she brushed her own teeth, she remembered the years of brushing his. She would eat and remember when she fed him. She'd pray to God at night for her strength not to fail and remember the prayers for her son to live another day. The shock of holding his body as the fire truck sirens blared towards the house changed who she was. Some of her friends understood that. Those were the friends she moved away from and rarely saw again.

My parents' time had been so consumed by my brother's needs that they both struggled to feel content in the additional 'free time' they had after his death. In Larned, Mom invested in quilting, a skill many of the women in her group had given untold hours to while raising their own children. Dad's mother, my grandmother Carol, had made at least one blanket for each of her eight children and each of her eighteen grandchildren. As the oldest granddaughter, I have a grandma Carol quilt from my infancy, my high school graduation and my wedding. Mom admired Grandma Carol's artistry in quilting.

However, after Dustin passed, mom's strongest years had passed too. Myotonic dystrophy had weakened Mom's grip. She constantly asked for help in opening peanut butter and pickle jars. Mom had sewn and crocheted for many years, and when I would craft with her in grade school, she operated scissors as well as anyone else. Age forty-nine was different. Cutting quilting blocks was difficult and threading a needle sometimes painful. Over the course of a year, Mom made a quilt for me with Bethany College Swede blue and yellow in square blocks and a personal message of love hand-sewn on the back. She tried to make Dad a quilt in the same way, with fabric of fishing scenes. She worked on it for over a year, restarted, cried in frustration, and simplified the project to adapt to her decreasing manual dexterity.

The quilting club was supportive, but her decreasing ability felt embarrassing and hard to explain. While she gained skill and experience, she was losing muscle control in a slow, almost unnoticeable way. It must have been exasperating to know she was less physically coordinated at age fifty than she was at age fifteen. Hobbies were frustrating for Mom. People observing from the outside, even those in her family, couldn't grapple with the depth of why it was so hard to do something for fun with a group of other women. She never blamed her MMD. I wonder if she recognized or accepted the connection. Was it too embarrassing to admit? Would anyone have understood if she told them?

Mom persisted, passively accepted her limitations, and made friends in her quilting group. She invited me to one of their annual year-end events where the quilters could display their recent projects and get a quilting pack of new ideas. Mom was proud enough of what she had done to display her work but told me she was embarrassed knowing other women had much more skill. She introduced me to many women who cared about her life. She asked me what kind of quilt Eli might like. Despite all the difficulties and frustrations, Mom found comfort and friendship in the quilting group.

Quilting is expensive. To expand her social circle and fuel her hobby, Mom wanted to work in Larned. It had been a few years since she had held a full time job.

Mom applied to a few places. With restrictions on how much she could lift or how long she could stand and no recent work experience or in-town references, she was overlooked. Her facial muscles had begun to visibly droop, giving her a tired appearance. She often was tired, in part due to myotonic dystrophy's effect of making it harder to sleep well and wake well-rested. She had to wear a medical sleeve on her leg to reduce swelling. She swayed with a limp in her gait. Dad told me more than once in these years that Mom would be in a wheelchair soon enough from her progressively worsening lower body state.

Her shoulders slouched, her eye contact was diminished, and she sat more often than stood. Mom had a shock of light grey hair in a stripe on the right side of her bangs. Her body was aging at a rapid pace, an irrevocable path silently propelled by her genetic code.

Being a car hop at Sonic delivering food to the cars was not ideal but was one of the only jobs available. Mom wanted a job which wouldn't be too physically strenuous. Raw need for social interaction, resignation from rejection by other potential employers, and growing isolation led her to try the job anyway. She'd been a good waitress and made friends working in restaurants, but this time she came home crying in the first week of work.

She had carried a tray of four slushies, lost her balance, steadied herself on a pole with her right hand, and spilled the drinks. The customers weren't mean; her boss didn't lecture. She just felt so helpless. She thought she could barely keep herself steady while walking, much less contribute to excellent customer service and speedy deliveries. Mom wasn't fast or surefooted.

She wanted to quit. Dad wanted her instead to work only mornings. Mom called me to talk it over. The conversation went something like this:

"Hi, hun, have time to talk?"

"Sure, Mom. How has your day been?"

"Oh, it was... pretty good." Her voice lagged on "pretty". I waited, but she didn't elaborate.

"I'm glad to hear you had a good day. I've been working on a term paper. If I didn't have practice, I don't think I would have gotten outside today."

"It's nice to get outside. I get outside with my job."

"Today was hot! At softball practice, running in the outfield for so long, I really wore myself out."

"You're taking on a lot right now with planning a wedding, classes, softball, and substitute teaching." Her voice became warmer: she enjoyed trying to take care of me. "Are you drinking enough water to keep up your energy?"

I laughed a bit. "Yes, Mother. I'm drinking lots of water. You taught me well."

She didn't reply. Dad had told me she wanted to quit her job at Sonic. I wanted to talk to her about her job and the heat, but I didn't want to seem like I thought I knew better than her. I led into it gently.

"I remember when I would go work at Sonic during high school after classes and practice. That job wasn't easy." I waited, then continued. "How's the Sonic in Larned treating you?"

"Oh, it's nice. I get out of the house and get to talk to people, but I do get so tired."

"It's not the easiest job to be a car hop."

"I know, especially on hot days. But it's all I could find. No one is hiring in Larned."

"Yeah, rough market in a small town right now."

"Your dad has a good job, though. He loves helping his brother. His nephews were out working with him this week, too."

"It's nice that Dad gets to be so connected in Larned." I hesitated. "What about you? Think anyone at work could grow to be a friend?"

She gave a deep sigh. "No, Darcy. The young girls at work think I'm an idiot. I'm slow, so they can do two orders when I do one. Somehow I was short when I counted my cash at the end of the day. I know I made tips. I didn't even have enough money to meet my sales. I had to give some of my own money."

I paused a second. I didn't want anyone to take advantage of Mom, but I didn't know anyone she worked with. "Mom, be careful. That might not have been your fault."

"I'm sure it was. I spilled drinks the other day. I got someone's order wrong today. I can barely think in the heat." Her voice cracked. "I just feel so stupid."

"Mom, you're not stupid. You're learning a new job."

"I've done waitressing before and been good at it. I just... I can't... voice, I can't voca..."

There was a muffled noise through the phone. Mom had developed a habit: when she slurred her speech or when she couldn't remember the right word, which was more and more often, she would slap herself in the mouth then try to start over. I cringed.

"It's okay if you can't vocalize as well with your coworkers now. I mean, they're younger, a different generation."

"No, Darcy! It's because I'm just not good at it. I'm not good at any of it. I can't count money, I can't walk straight, and no one wants me to work with them because I just slow them down." Her words came with the sound of saliva. I imagined the tears on her face.

"Maybe you can study for the test to be a cook and stay inside. You could..."

She cut me off. "I can't do that. I come home and sleep after work. They won't want me to move up and get paid more; they barely want me to work there. I'm slow!"

In a family with genetic disease and a special education history, "slow" is a loaded word. She meant more about herself than her speed.

I leveraged Dad's idea to try to offer hope. "If you worked half days you would be fresher, maybe even faster?"

She gasped for air and composure. Asthma was making breathing, talking, and crying hard to do simultaneously. "Oh, I suppose."

She didn't say anything else, and for a moment neither did I. I thought part of it may be that she felt betrayed, that she realized I had talked to Dad when I made the same suggestion he had.

She asked in a pained voice: "Are you disappointed in me?"

"No. No, Mom, I'm not. You don't have to work. The bills are paid."

"Yeah, by your dad's retirement check, but, with the car he bought so I'd be comfortable and saving to visit New Mexico to make me happy, I don't have money to go do things. I just stay in the house then. It's lonely staying in the house. It's not about the money, Darcy. I want to be able to do things, talk to people. I don't want to stay home and use Dad's money."

"Half days wouldn't be so bad. You could get out and talk and not have to work through the heat..."

I heard the defeat in her voice. With resignation she said, "Yeah, it wouldn't be so bad. But then --"

"What is it, Mom?"

"Then they'll have to hire someone else anyway, and why would they keep me? I don't even know if I could make it four hours without spilling a drink. And some of the girls, they aren't nice about it. They just want me out of their way."

I was at a loss for words. I knew employment in small town Kansas was hard. Mom didn't have many options. She probably didn't relate well to a younger generation of car hops. And even if she did relate well, she wasn't trying to get out of the house to find pity – she wanted to find self-worth. I didn't think it was going to happen through Sonic.

"Maybe half days would get enough money to…"

"It's not the money!"

"Hey, I'm not trying to make you angry, okay?"

"You don't understand. You almost never come to Larned. It's different here."

"I'm pretty busy as a college athlete, Mom. I'm sorry."

"It's not your fault." She cried audibly, wheezing with her tears. "I need to go. I love you."

"I love you too, Mom. I'm sorry it's hard."

"It's okay. I have a new puzzle I'm going to do. I'll call you tomorrow."

I pictured my mother home alone as Dad worked, dejected from failure at attempts to be part of the working community of Larned and not having another easy way in. "Bye, Mom. I love you."

She hung up. I buried my face in my hands and let a few tears fall. She wanted out of the house to earn some extra money to spend on a social hobby and talk to people. Instead she felt shame. The waitress who met her husband while serving tables three years after competing in Miss Otero County now felt like an inept car hop people shunned rather than sought.

As Mom's disease progressed, her pronunciation suffered. This impeded phone conversations. I wanted to be a supportive daughter, listen, and help her find meaning in her day to day activities. I wanted to tell her about my life's joys and ask her advice on becoming a mother. I wanted her to feel that she had raised me well and deserved my time. Unfortunately, I wasn't great at it. I couldn't always understand her, which sometimes led to feigned listening, unrelated answers, or too many questions about what she said.

Mom needed someone to talk to. Besides Dad, I was her most important personal contact. Her decreasing ability to communicate and the two hour drive put a gap in our once-close relationship. On top of that, I was young and naïve and still thought that women had to find empowerment through self-actualization, willpower, and positive attitude. On the phone, I didn't nurture Mom's hurt feelings. I didn't understand her growing insecurity over her decreasing capabilities. She heard 'work harder,' 'advocate for yourself to your boss,' 'write down small goals to become better at work,' or 'purposefully try to talk to your coworkers to build relationships.' I gave her advice towards empowerment in the phase of her life where she was least empowered, when she was losing control of an ailing body.

Mom fought a terminal disease, one that ate at her muscles and in turn nibbled away at her self-confidence, her security, and her reputation. She did not wear a sign that said 'victim of genetic misfortune,' nor would she want that label. She did not elicit pity or the type of friendly smiles Dustin drew in his wheelchair. Her disease was hidden, and when it charged forward, taking over her body, she drew back into further social isolation.

Mom worked part time at Sonic for a while. Eventually, she felt too worn out to continue a struggle where rewards seemed so small. Why should she fight her body and her emotions to socialize with people that she felt she burdened? Why should she struggle past the insecurities to buy fabric for a craft she didn't have the manual dexterity to excel at? Mom gracefully put in her two weeks' notice and finished out the time as a woman who genuinely wanted to do her best and be meaningful. Then she slid back into the obscurity of a reclusive housewife with no long-term social ties in a small town and no children in an area where the best entertainment is the hometown football game.

I tried to talk with Mom every day. But, a few months after the Sonic phone call, I could barely understand her on the phone. I was busy and felt like we talked about the same things. She could tell I enjoyed the phone calls less and less, so she called less and less – another layer of increasing isolation. Dad told me my phone calls brightened my mother's day. A phone call wasn't too much effort, but often enough I let myself be "too busy" to do it. My abilities and pace of life led me to choices that also isolated Mom.

Mom did try to work again, this time as a substitute paraprofessional in the local school district. She had been a full-time paraprofessional in 1992 in San Antonio, Texas. She had loved it then, and talked at home about the good in her work. While her time in San Antonio inspired me as a child to also want to work in education, her run with the Larned district lacked luster. Mom's heart was in it, but one day in a grade school class, during a long period of down time, Mom fell asleep. Mom would fall asleep five minutes into a car ride and during many movies, slept more than ten hours most days, and preferred to have an afternoon nap when she could. Severe fatigue is a major problem for approximately one third of those with adult onset myotonic dystrophy MMD. Excessive sleepiness is common for women like my mother. The teacher didn't know Mom's medical history or the common symptoms. It may not have mattered anyway.

A school district doesn't have to fire a substitute or even give a reason why the district no longer calls. The phone calls just stop. Mom knew she had made a mistake. She blamed herself, begrudged her body for betraying her heart. She didn't tell me about the experience on the phone; she waited until I visited her house for dinner. By that time our phone conversations often ended in tears because she couldn't help me understand her.

She cried when she told me about falling asleep. She talked using her hands. She slapped herself in the face when she couldn't get the right word out. She asked, "Do you think they'll call me again?"

"Well, it's a small town. If lots of people get sick, they might need a sub."

"Yea, but they are making cuts in the district. They might not even have para-subs next year." Her eyes were bleary. She knew her employment options were limited, and somewhere in the unspoken murmurs of her heart, she knew this was role she once made meaningful impact in with a full time job. "I didn't mean to fall asleep. The teacher just didn't give me anything to do. She talked so long."

I wish I had more wisdom in that moment to give her a better response. I told her, "The teacher can't see what you meant to do. She saw you were asleep. She's worried about the kids' work ethic. It wasn't personal that she told you she would be talking to the office about it."

'It wasn't personal.' Those were dumb words to say. Of course it was personal. Mom was trying to mean something to someone in Larned, felt that she failed, and wouldn't get the chance again. It was intensely personal. It tipped the edge of her self-confidence in contributing meaningfully to society through work. She did get a few more substitute calls after that, but the calls were rare. She replied positively every time. None of those phone calls were from the grade school, though. It wasn't much of a job at that point, and each time she went in insecure, worried that her body's increasing weakness might betray her, that her actions wouldn't match her intent because she was so often sleepy.

That substituting job was the last one she ever worked.

Chapter 8
Give Kids the World

One of the only times Mom met another woman who had passed a terminal genetic disease on to a child was in 1997 in Kissimmee, Florida, thanks to the Give Kids the World Village and the Make a Wish Foundation. The wish team that visited our home on Hill Air Force Base, Utah, spent many hours with the family. Two female volunteers had the job of meeting Dustin and discovering his one true wish. The catch was in accessing the 'one true wish' of an eight-year-old boy who couldn't speak. Honestly, they could have brought him ice cream and he would have thought it grand. My parents talked to the wish team about Dustin, what he liked, his medical history, health restrictions that might limit what he could do, etc. Dad suggested at one point that we could go on a trip to Atlanta and watch the Braves play and meet Greg Maddux. He may have meant it as a joke, but such a suggestion sent up a red flag for the wish granters. They wondered what interest Dustin had in Greg Maddux. Indeed, it was not his interest Dad mentioned, but mine. Dad told the wish team that the only thing they had to do to make Dustin think it was a perfect day was to buy him a balloon, Cheetos, and a Mountain Dew.

Dad was often like that. I think he felt he couldn't give me enough time or that he invested so much more of his efforts and money into Dustin. He would splurge for me on old Braves baseball cards from the 1950s, take me on a monthly trip to play laser tag with friends, coach my softball teams, and stretch the budget to buy me a Lego set 'just because.'

Our real suggestion was that Dustin would love Disney World because his favorite toys were his Disney puppets of Mickey, Minnie, Pluto, Winnie the Pooh, and Barney. The wish team visited a second time though, trying to make sure they knew what Dustin, not Darcy, wished for.

To convince them that Dustin's wish was for Disney World, I brought in Dustin's Winnie the Pooh and Pluto puppets and started a mock conversation. Dustin immediately raised his head and set in motion. I handed out puppets. Dad got Mickey, Mom got Minnie, and Pluto and Barney went to the two wish granters.

Mom had the most experience playing puppets with Dustin. She brought Minnie close to Dustin's face, made a "boop," and closed the puppet fingers on his nose. Dustin chortled in joy. Mom ran Minnie behind Dustin's ear to kiss his head. Dustin turned to look at Minnie, smiled with a slobbery grin, and hissed in excitement.

Dad stood in front of Dustin, raising Mickey high. He flexed his fingers in and out, as if Mickey were a spider, and said playfully, "Mickey's going to get you; he's gonna get you!" Dustin's head whipped to Dad so quickly that he had to rebalance his upper body with his arms. He relaxed his neck so that the back of his head rested on his back. He laughed hysterically and pointed to Mickey. The puppet grabbed Dustin's hand and wiggled.

I glanced at our guests. Dustin's eyes followed mine, and he pointed to his favorite puppet, Barney. Dustin grunted, indicating he wanted the puppet near. He turned his palm to an open hand, pulling his fingers toward the base of his thumb repeatedly in his sign for "want."

The wish team member beamed a genuinely accepting smile and came over to Dustin. In her best purple dinosaur voice, she said "Hello, I'm Barney." Dustin scooted right next to her leg. "If you'd like, you can meet me this summer in Florida. Would you enjoy that?"

He grabbed her arm and pulled Barney to his chest, where he embraced her and the puppet with both arms. The next time she visited our house was to tell us the details of our trip and share the news that not only did we get an all-expense paid trip, with a stay in the Give Kids the World village, but that we'd have the spending cash and a personal gift from her, a small Mickey Mouse stuffed animal to take on the trip.

She told me before she left that she was glad to see that what made Dustin most happy was to see his family relaxed and joyful with him. She said she was happy that this trip would give us, as his caretakers, some of the reward that we deserved. She'd seen the pure joy of Dustin's life – a boy uncomplicated by competition, deceit, or popularity.

The gifting power of the Make a Wish Foundation is awe-inspiring, an impressive pooling of volunteers, networking, and benevolent hearts. The trip was an amazing opportunity we never would have taken without the Make a Wish Foundation. Besides helicopters flying to hospitals, this was Dustin's first trip on a plane. It was certainly my first trip where we had five hundred dollars available. They gave us the money in cash and didn't ask for receipts. My family had a habit of living frugally. While we bought souvenirs, including a Goofy hat and watch for me, Disney World t-shirts at Wal-Mart, and food, we made it home with over one hundred dollars. Perhaps the greatest benefit, though, was finding a "village" of people in similar situations, in which a rare disease feels less lonely.

Give Kids the World Village is a huge seventy-acre, nonprofit resort near all the major Disney attractions in Florida where children with life-threatening illnesses and their families are treated to weeklong, free fantasy vacations. We were lodged and fed in the Village for free. I played with other kids like me or my brother for hours in the free arcade. Nightly entertainment was scheduled to enrich the lives on some very special kids and their blessed families – all for free. The restaurant was staffed by volunteers, and no tips were accepted. The whole Village was built to serve these special families and give them a week to remember the rest of their lives.

The Give Kids the World Village was a special place, but as an eleven-year-old girl, I wanted all the action and adventure I could get at the Disney parks, the Magic Kingdom, Epcot Center, and Disney's Hollywood Studios. With Dustin in a wheelchair, we had the equivalent of a "fast pass," even if Dustin didn't ride. Dad rode with me on Splash Mountain four times, I rode the Tower of Terror three times, and we went on the Space Mountain roller coaster twice. We watched parades and firework shows. Dustin cuddled with a pretty lady dressed as Ariel from the Little Mermaid. Whenever Dustin saw a character he recognized, he would extend his legs in excitement, hiss or giggle, point the way, and start pushing his wheels that direction. The Disney parks were special, and many of our best memories are on that trip to Disney, but the true gift, the part of the experience hardest to duplicate, was Mom's chance to meet other women like her.

Mom stood next to Dustin while he rode the Give Kids the World carousel, read books to him at the Village house we stayed in, and chatted with other mothers who carried a gene they passed on to their terminally ill children. She savored the slower paced world of parents who, for a rare moment in a life in which their child faces life threatening illness every day, could forget about all the other cares in the world and just enjoy being with others like them. Mom would have been content staying all five days in that utopian Village. She didn't have to fight crowds or lines, climb stairs, or endure the sunny summer sun. People there had a similar background and some intimately understood the burdens of being both caretaker and victim of a genetic disease.

The Village catered to families with limited mobility or who couldn't easily spend a day at a Disney park and have energy left over. The pace of life there was Dustin's pace, her pace, a different pace. While I wanted to ride the Tower of Terror as many times as possible, Mom found a home in the Village. While I yearned for excitement and amusement, Mom wanted to stay in this whimsical village of mushroom-shaped buildings purposely and compassionately created to be a sanctuary for those who for whom life sped by too quickly.

In the Village Mom found a gift better than the most entertaining amusement park. She found acceptance, recognition of her struggles, women she could relate to, children she felt sympathy for, families like ours, families worse off than ours, and families that would bless ours. People often offered us compassion but rarely understood our family, particularly Mom. Mom's hopes and aspirations weren't for the typical American dream. That Village, with its fairy tale themed architecture and décor, provided an escape from American materialism and the personal competitions and let Mom feel connected to those around her. Mom wanted to enjoy the solace and community of people like her, those who didn't value awards, achievements, and entertainment as much as contentment.

Mom lived each day with Dustin like a gift, not something to use only in building some type of stepping stone but another chance to be with her terminally ill son and enjoy her own health. I didn't understand that at age eleven. Dustin's time was limited. I wish I had been wise enough to recognize Mom's was, too. It was fun to ride down Splash Mountain or drop down the Tower of Terror, but it wasn't life altering; it didn't renew my soul. The Give the Kids the World Village gave that opportunity to Mom, helped renew her faith in society by giving her a community, however temporary, of people like her in a situation similar to ours. That Village is a blessing because of the acceptance and openness it can create through philanthropy and good will.

Chapter 9
Social Ladders

Openness and acceptance were easier to find in the Give Kids the World Village than middle school, where I had to learn the demographics of the athletics social ladder. The summer between my seventh and eighth grade year we moved from Mom's home town of Alamogordo, New Mexico, closer to Dad's family in Salina, Kansas. The first athletic opportunity available to me in middle school was volleyball.

Dad took me to Play It Again Sports to buy knee pads. I often ended up on the ground and wanted the best protection I could get so I found a white pair with a thick padded shield. My bulky, uncool, obviously used knee protected me from bruises with the tradeoff of attracting ridicule.

Athleticism was my only advantage in a sport I'd never played. I ran hard every lap, passing stragglers in our five minute run, letting everyone get a good look at my hand-me-down shorts many sizes too big. After our run we huddled around our coach, who was seven months pregnant. One popular and talented girl who competed in beauty pageants looked around at all the players and said, "We must have had a tough workout. I smell sweat." Her eyes scanned the players, her lips curled into the smile of middle school cruelty. "And blood."

Her eyes locked on mine. She grinned. Another girl laughed. The two looked at each other and giggled again. They were on the inside. I wasn't.

Our pregnant coach struggled with her proximity to our sweaty huddle. She said, "Yes, I smell it too. I can't… I need to leave. Wendy, finish up the huddle." The girls laughed some more. Uncertain, I giggled too.

Gathering my school clothes in the locker room, one of the more gentle girls, a quiet and friendly person, came to me and said,

"Darcy, you might want to change before you get in the car." She smiled and shrugged as I stared at her, trying to comprehend.

My blank stare brought her to explain. "You have a spot on your shorts." She smiled kindly and left.

I checked. I had bled through my shorts.

The girls had been laughing at me. I was the smell of blood. I was the reason my coach couldn't stay in the huddle.

I felt isolated. I wished Mom had more time to teach me about fashion and hygiene. Dad should never have let me get that bad haircut. Why did I have to wear my aunt's old shorts to volleyball practice? It wasn't easy to fit in.

With all the energy my family spent in taking care of Dustin, I knew our family valued different things than many families. I felt low, like being Dustin's sister and having parents who worked hard to meet our needs didn't put me on the same social standing as those girls. They had resources in abundance, time and money to wear the latest fashions, and mothers who got monthly perms or color treatments. Mom didn't have time to read fashion magazines or time in the morning routine to do my hair. Those girls didn't know Dustin, Mom or much about me, but they knew I had a spot on my shorts. It took a while to make friends on the team.

By the time I was a sophomore in high school, I had found acceptance with the upper class ethos that dominated high school athletics. I worked hard, was athletic, listened, and didn't complain. However, my parents still worked the night shift at Wal-Mart, wore ten-year-old clothes that rarely got ironed, didn't wear makeup or cologne, and pushed around a handicapped kid who made awkward noises at important parts of the game.

Did my teammates accept me and my family? By the time I was an upperclassman, certainly. The girls I played with for four years loved my brother, knew my parents by name, and thought I was one of the luckiest kids at Central High School to have such a loving family.

My sophomore year wasn't easy, though. My strategy to try harder than anyone else stirred up the same type of animosity from the juniors and seniors my 'new kid' eighth grade year did.

During one van ride in particular two varsity players wanted to pass along some advice. They wanted to help me "fit in." I sat in the back seat, the two girls sat in the row ahead of me, and Coach drove. After some whispering and texting, the two girls started a mock conversation, pretending to talk about an opposing player.

"Did you see that girl's mustache? I didn't see it at first, but, standing at the net, it's hard not to notice. I felt so bad for her." The taller girl spoke in her best 'let's go talk to the Indians' pretend voice. Right away I knew something was off.

"Yeah. She is a pretty girl otherwise. But it's hard to like her with a mustache. Doesn't she know there are things she can do about that?"

The other girl responded with excessive enthusiasm. "It isn't even that rare for a girl to have a mustache. My mom has to take care of hers."

"Really? Is it hard? What does she do to take care of it?" I slouched my shoulders and pretended to be asleep. Mom and I both had slight mustaches. I did what I saw her do – pluck it occasionally and go on with the more important things in life. I didn't want confrontation with the girls. I'd rather pretend I was oblivious.

"Well, she uses cream, or plucks it. That can hurt sometimes, but it doesn't cost much."

"I heard there is surgery to remove unwanted facial hair. But that is like five hundred dollars."

"Yeah. That's expensive. It's not hard for a girl to not have facial hair, though. She can always just shave it for free."

It was pragmatic advice, and as an independent adult with a professional job, I'm better now at managing what nature gave me. Mom gave more attention to her grooming when she was younger. But with two kids, one of them in a wheelchair, her time was much more limited. She accepted her looks and gave her decision-making power to more vital issues. I wished I had her strength to focus on what mattered.

I was mortified. It wasn't like I didn't try to control my looks. I plucked, but it hurt and took forever. I bought the cream, but it was expensive to use regularly. I shaved, but stubby hairs reappeared quickly. I didn't have a good answer. Why should I even care? My facial hair didn't matter at home where pneumonia, surgeries, and loving on Dustin took precedence. But it mattered to those girls who could see my face from across the net. My world was different than theirs, and the girls' perceptions made me insecure. I wanted to be accepted by the girls on the varsity team. It wasn't easy.

While this evolving social awareness was valuable, thinking my family didn't fit the traditional American lifestyle came with consequences. I had to battle being embarrassed about how my parents appeared at volleyball games. Part of me didn't want my teammates around Dustin to see him slobber on hand-me-down clothes. I wanted the girls to know I was smart and capable. I wanted them to value me without judging my family. Mostly, I wanted to fit in with my teammates from more typical families.

One of the girls who pointed out the intricacies of facial hair maintenance had a mother she closely resembled: tall and beautiful, with well-rounded shoulders, dark, well-maintained hair, and attractive, expensive clothing. Her mother hosted team dinners, brought snacks, took pictures to post online, and stopped to talk to my family after games. She talked to all the families after games. She was socially successful and charismatic.

When she talked to my family, she didn't hug my brother or say how cute he was. Not everyone did, but after what her daughter said in the van, I wondered how she perceived my mother and her barely-visible upper lip hair. What ran through her head as she exchanged pleasantries with Mom, clad in her Wal-Mart employee work shirt with the iconic 'roll-back prices' smiley face?

Did this woman secretly desire to give Mom advice on how to be socially acceptable like her daughter did for me? Was she offended by the hair visible on Mom's lip? The two women had similar hair color and similar eye brows. Was she ever seen in public with even the slightest trace of facial hair? How much free time did she have at home to worry about hair and makeup compared to Mom? Would she have gotten along with Mom if they had met before Mom's disease began to progress?

Mom's hair was in a loose pony tail with curly wisps escaping above her ears. The other mom's dark hair had no frizz and curled gently under her ears, dancing with her dangling earrings. Mom wore no jewelry or makeup. She had shifted her graveyard sleep schedule to make my volleyball game and had bags under her eyes. My parents stood out in the volleyball crowd.

My parents dressed differently, cared about different things, conversed in a different set of pleasantries. If I had another teammate on free lunches, I didn't know it. I wasn't ashamed of my parents. However, I wanted to make my own way in the world. I wanted to be able to do things my parents weren't able to because life dealt them a different set of cards. To do that I thought I had to work hard on my own.

I invested seriously in being a top student and strong athlete. My focus was narrow and funneled on building future success. It was distracting when Dustin made a funny noise in the middle of a match and my teammates giggled and told me how cute he was. I didn't want to talk to my parents between matches; I wanted to focus on the next game. I didn't want to go sit with my parents when waiting for the next match. Oftentimes I'd let them sit alone, on the edge where they thought Dustin was least distracting, and try to seem busy with my teammates or warming up. In my school involvements, I didn't want to focus on my parents. I wanted to focus on learning skills my parents didn't have the resources to teach.

Luckily, I had a kind and compassionate coach, Mrs. Lisa Evers, who saw past the game. After one game Dad brought me a Gatorade and granola bar.

"Thanks Dad." I said simply. I took the food and drink and left my parents to go eat by some teammates. My parents stood there and watched my back as I walked away.

Coach Evers observed the scene. After I finished my snack, she called me to her. "Darcy, you have some of the most supportive parents on the team. They've been to every game, even traveling."

I looked at her, waiting for her point.

"Your parents make many sacrifices for you. You know, it's okay if you talk to them at meets. Sports are about family too."

I smiled at her. I was getting permission to do something. That wasn't bad.

Then she was frank: "You should show them more appreciation when they come to your games. It isn't easy for parents to be at as many events as they are. They really want to support you."

I dropped my head. I understood. I didn't know what to say. I nodded. "Yes ma'am." Blood ran to my cheeks in shame.

I was angry at first. It hurt to hear, but I'm glad she called me out on my behavior. I was offended that she thought I didn't appreciate my parents just because of what she saw when I was trying to focus. I wanted to tell her I was trying to make something of myself – that I had to work extra hard to beat the odds that face families with genetic disease. I even wanted to tell her that I had to use my time while I was young, just in case I carried the disease like Mom did. I wanted to tell her off. I didn't.

Instead, the next game they came to, I talked to my parents between matches. I asked them about their day, how work went, what Dustin did in school. I told them about my day. I sat down next to them in the stands. I looked over at my coach, who was starting to round up the players. She smiled when we met eyes. She cared more about me than just my performance on her team. As a typical sibling in an atypical family, it can be easy to get stuck on building skill independently to find a new way of life instead of enjoying and appreciating family. My coach helped me open my focus to appreciate what I had at the same time I was building for my future.

Even when they worked the graveyard shift, my parents came to almost every one of my volleyball, basketball and softball games in high school and college. My parents were my constant supporters. I'm glad someone had the courage to tell me to appreciate my family's attendance more when I was young.

Mom even helped me when I refused to try. My senior year she brought home an application for a nationwide Wal-Mart scholarship program for children of employees. I took one look at the ten-page application packet and told her, "I have no chance, mom. There are too many applicants for me to win."

Mom asked me to complete the application for another few days, and each time I told her I was too busy, that it wasn't worth the time. The scholarship application gave her job a chance to matter more to my education and offered a chance to help pay for my schooling. It mattered to her, and I treated it like a waste of my effort.

A few days before the application was due, after the packet had sat on the kitchen table for upwards of two weeks, Mom filled in everything she could without me on that ten-page application.

"Darcy, I started this for you. Do you want to finish it? My boss says you'd have a good chance." She smiled in a way that looked slightly self-conscious, in an obvious attempt to persuade and charm as her cheeks creased in on themselves and she tilted her head slightly to the right.

I was wearing my backpack over my sweaty practice shirt. "I still haven't changed Mom. I have a lot of homework tonight. I don't think I can."

"But it won't take you much time now. There are only a few blank spots left."

I flipped through the application packet to see how much she had done.

"Here I didn't know what to put. I left that part blank, but I filled in all your activities I could remember all the way back to middle school."

I glanced over the list. It had an impressive span; Mom recorded things I had long ago forgotten. "I went back through your box of awards to do it. I've kept all of them in your box in the basement. There isn't much left, and I'll help you fill it out if you'd like."

I met her eyes and grinned when she smiled at me and shrugged her shoulders in a questioning way. She cared so much.

"Yeah, Mom. I can finish this. How about we fill it out right here?" We sat together, and I answered the rest of the questions. I finished the application, thinking I had done my duty as a busy daughter by placating my mother. I didn't think I had a chance at the scholarship, but at least had finally sat down to spend time with Mom to do something she wanted for me. Mom had taken that ten-page application and turned it into a personal endeavor to give a gift from mother to daughter.

Later, Mom informed me with pride that I had won a four year renewable scholarship for $2,000 a year. The honor was announced in front of all her coworkers during a work meeting. She beamed with pride and bragged to all her friends. She never told anyone, 'Yeah, and I filled out seventy percent of it for the lazy bum.'

Mom told me I deserved it, that I was the kind of student who could win a national award and the kind of girl capable of anything. Mom loved me, and her persistence, more than my ability or initiative, was going to pay for a good share of my education. Mom provided well for me. My ability to be economically mobile and live a stable life is in large part due to her reading to me every night when I was young, going on summer softball trips as a sponsor, attending every high school event possible, and doing the little things for me that I was too blind or stubborn to do. God bless those efforts; she did a good job.

Chapter 10
Numb and Angry

Isaiah 55:8-9 of the Bible says, "'For my thoughts are not your thoughts, neither are your ways my ways,' declares the LORD. 'As the heavens are higher than the earth, so are my ways higher than your ways and my thoughts than your thoughts.'"(NIV)

When Dustin died, Mom, Dad, and I had been taking care of him and trying to prolong his life for years. The sudden severity of someone coming to the end of their life is jarring in finality. It's easy to feel angry when what you prepare the way for isn't what is meant to be. When I lost Dustin, I was sixteen. In the first few days after he passed, it was 'easy' to go about with what others perceive as strength. During those days I felt needed, as if my hardiness could bolster the durability of my family members. Each day was a clear mile marker of the success of surviving after a loved one's death. When Dustin passed away, I wanted to be strong for my parents.

Of course I cried, but there were many times in front of people when hard discussions were met with dry eyes and a stoic tone. At sixteen, my life would go on. I looked forward to college. I tried to love my parents through showing them how successful they had been in raising me by doing my best in everything I could. I wanted to show them they succeeded by being successful even after Dustin's death.

Behind closed doors I wept, I wrote, and I threw things in anger. I questioned God. I pleaded to know why He would give me something so beautiful, take it away, and leave me to the rest of the world with an entertainment based culture of gluttony and selfish desire. I didn't know what to think of heaven, I couldn't make sense of people's purpose here on Earth, and I was mad at God for making Dustin's life so short. Dustin was so beautifully different from the corrupted world he was born into. God's ways weren't my ways, and that concept led to resentment. Alone in my room, I asked God, "Why are you such a cruel puppeteer?"

This anger rarely bubbled to a public surface. I thought people needed me to be strong. Dustin was a beacon of hope, someone people could look at and get a glimpse of God's love through how he embraced simple joys. In my mind, I had to show the outside world how visible strength and faith had been built in my life through God's giving my family a blessing that appeared as a challenge. Part of me thought Dustin was in my life so that I could be special too – that I was born to be resilient and stronger by my family's trials. I tried to maintain the type of hope Dustin gave others simply by living, and I refused to acknowledge the full pain of the loss. I walked the high school halls after Dustin's death numbly, buffering myself from feeling. I expressed little emotion, even in times where my coaches wanted me to celebrate to raise team morale. I lost myself in goals and tasks so I wouldn't have to feel the moment or let emotions drive the situation. I wrote journal entries during history lectures -- not complaining, not disrupting, just drifting along with compliance and enough aptitude to get by. It was my worst academic year.

When I couldn't ignore the world by writing in my journal, sometimes I escaped the classroom. One person in the building had worked with me every year since eighth grade, my gifted counselor Kay Schiebler. She had been to Dustin's funeral and kept me afloat at school by letting me talk, or cry, in her office anytime I needed. She saved me from breaking down in public or skipping school. She helped me process the hardest year of my schooling.

I drifted emotionally as the proximity of Dustin's death faded in the minds of others. The "I have to be strong" buffer wore out. I had a boyfriend who wrote a poem and gave me a cat after Dustin passed away. He turned out to be a compulsive liar who spent hours on questionable websites. After I broke up with him, I dated a pilot student who enticed me into skipping school, lying to my basketball coach, and going to an Evanescence concert. Later he changed his major because of bad grades, didn't seem like he knew what he wanted, and partied with other girls as if he weren't in a relationship. Dating older guys while trying to figure out where to go with life my senior year didn't endow the wisdom I must have been looking for. Fear of my future began to overwhelm my stoic chasing of success.

I caught part of "The Breakfast Club" on TV. It had a one-liner that spurred my search for self into rebellion: "Do you always do what you're told, sporto?" Shortly after watching only part of "The Breakfast Club," I quit my high school softball team with two weeks left in the season.

I'd been a coach pleaser through three sports for almost four years. I was team captain. I'd never publicly argued with a coach, and I rarely complained. My decision surprised everyone.

I had told Mom in the car the day before I quit that I feared my emotions toward my coach. It was too strong of an emotion to come to hate someone who I felt was disrespecting who I was and where I was in life. I couldn't explain exactly why my coach didn't like me, but I felt small and irksome when she would speak to me. Mom said I needed to talk to the coach about what had happened the day before. After I jogged -- rather than sprinted -- to the right fielder's missed ball in practice, Coach reprimanded me. I deserved it. My coach probably liked me just fine, but I didn't like the emotions I was feeling. I didn't need it.

I called the coach three times after that practice and finally left a message. The day I quit, I went her office before we left to try to talk to her in person about the event and how disrespected I felt. She told me, "I don't talk to players about issues like that" and ended the conversation. My emotions bubbled on the bus ride in a way I hadn't let them do in public for years.

I played the double header with more emotions coursing through me than thoughts. Calm, the emotion I'd survived on for over a year, evaded me. I was benched in the middle of the second game after I struck out twice. I let a tear drop in the dugout.

I went to my coach with angry eyes. I tried to ask calmly. "Why am I sitting on the bench?"

"You struck out twice. What do you think?" She boomed in response.

"It's a defensive inning. I've played every inning in centerfield the last three years." My voice wasn't as flat as I hoped.

"Well" Her attitude was obvious in her tone. "Maybe it's time for someone else to get the chance."

"Is this about what happened yesterday? You should have answered when I called." I heard my voice crack. "We need to talk about it."

"Now is not the time, Darcy. Sit down."

I felt more negative emotion than I had in all year. In public. I couldn't bottle it.

"If this is how I'm going to be treated to play softball, I'm going to leave."

She yelled her response. "Way to be the bigger person, Darcy!"

My stoicism would have crashed in a yelling match. I had to go. I don't know that I had many better options, but I tried to clear all emotion from my face. I tried not to feel anything. I walked away from her, picked up my bag, and asked my parents to take me home.

In the car, I balled. I told Mom I didn't want to hate my coach but that I felt I had to get away from the way she treated me. Dad didn't tell me I was wrong, but I could see his disappointment. My emotional endurance had run out, and it had just cost me my senior season in the sport I was best at.

I thought, "At least I kept my dignity and walked away without losing my temper or being hateful." I was supposed to go to college to play softball. I was risking my athletic future to try to avoid negative emotions. My coach was a good coach and kind person. It wasn't her fault, but I wasn't emotionally capable of handling everything I felt as high school was ending.

The athletic director called me into his office the next day. I didn't want to go. I didn't want to have to face the situation. He asked if I'd go back to the team to finish the last two weeks. He told me I had a good career at Central, that I should finish strong, and that my college coach wouldn't want me sitting out of the playoffs.

I listened to him, took my time to think, closed my eyes and breathed deeply. "No, I don't want to hate that woman. I'm not going to go back to seeing her every day."

He stared at me. I stared back with empty, detached eyes. If any emotion showed on my face, it wasn't because I chose to reveal it. It was easier to walk away than face the emotions for ten more days in a situation that hurt during a time I hurt too much.

Eventually, he asked me, "It's that simple, then? You're done?"

It wasn't that simple, but I just wanted it to be over. I wasn't out to pick a bigger fight; I was trying to be left alone. He pursed his lips, told me a story about coaching his own son and how they butted heads, and talked about how good athletes often have conflicts with coaches they have to work past. He gave me time to respond. I sat silently.

I tried to look him in the eyes. "I won't go back." I dropped my head in shame. "Not with her there. I can't feel that way."

Earlier in the year, I had asked for and received a letter of recommendation for college applications from my athletic director. He was one of the adults I respected most at the school. He drilled my eyes with his until I looked up at him.

His tone changed. He said simply, "I'm disappointed with you."

I didn't know what to say. I didn't want to feel it. I apologized and left.

I had tried so hard for the last year and a half to make high school a success. I wanted my parents to feel proud and successful with me. Part of my dignity dropped with the tears on his office floor. I had failed.

Later that week was Awards Night for the end of the academic year. When I sat down next to one of my best friends, she said, "No way, Darcy. As many awards as you will get tonight, I'm not sitting on the edge next to you and getting up every two minutes. You sit on the edge." I received a high number of award, and not getting one more shouldn't have hurt, but the one I didn't get represented my failure to be in control of my emotions: the Triple Crown Award for athletes who lettered in three sports in one academic year. I didn't get my third letter because I quit softball, because I refused to handle negative emotions, because I walked away after striking out. The athletic director handed out those awards.

The last award of the night was for the "Most Representative Senior Male and Female." I was one of the final three candidates. As I stood on stage with the other three candidates, with all the other students in attendance looking up at us, I felt proud. Standing on stage with lights and eyes on me for a big award, for a short second, I felt justified in quitting, as if I were the 'bigger person' my coach had mocked me with. Then I felt like a hypocrite, making everyone think I was strong and good when I was scared and angry and immature.

The Most Representative Senior Female award was first voted down to the final ten by the staff; then the students voted on the final ten to pick the winner. The voting finished shortly before I quit softball. I stood there thinking I was ashamed of who people thought I was versus who I felt like inside.

"And your 2004 Senior Most Representative Female is…. Darcy Bartz!"

The other two girls hugged me. I was told to step forward. From in front of the stage, one of my best friends said, "Darcy, don't look so embarrassed. You just won a great award!"

The whirlwind of emotions I couldn't control or escape were visible on my face in front of the whole crowd. Others said supportive things like "You look beautiful" or "You deserve this." I had earned the respect of my fellow students, but I wondered how many of them would have voted for me if that had happened after I quit the softball team. That night on that stage, after my name was announced, that is one of my most insecure moments in life. I didn't feel like I deserved the award.

My heart was pained by my own decision to walk away from my softball team. I had protected my emotions, and instead of dealing with adversity, I quit the team. I was more willing to damage my reputation and endanger my future as a college athlete than let myself feel emotions that weren't easy to control. I may have avoided hate or anger, but instead I felt deep shame and embarrassment.

In the first year after Dustin's passing, I survived by trying to be strong for others and ignoring my own feelings as much as possible. My senior year gave me more freedom: I dated again, and my emotions were akin to probably what most high school girls feel in the chaotic confusion of a young woman trying to figure out who she is. I repressed my emotions, and, instead of allowing myself to feel anger or even hatred, I made a choice which left me sad, ashamed, and embarrassed.

By award night, a month before high school ended, I had my tuition costs and more covered for Bethany College, a Christian college I was excited to attend. I was dating my future husband. Everything seemed to be going right. During my last week of high school I received many kind words from the students and staff, including a genuine compliment from my athletic director on how successful of a high school career I had. Nearly every time I was complimented though, I felt undeserving. Often I would reply, "Yeah, but I shouldn't have quit the softball team."

Without my brother, I felt I had to define myself not by my sibling, but by my success. I needed to make my parents proud, to be their strength, to carry on Dustin's message by being the person he helped build me to be. I was hard on myself, had standards too high to be realistic, and repressed a lot of real emotions to try to be something I wasn't: everything to everyone. I went through the last two weeks of my high school career feeling like a failure.

That year would have been easier if I talked to a therapist or discussed depression treatment with a doctor. Mentally I walked a dangerous path, and I would continue to have anger issues within, with God, and with my boyfriend. It took a long time to admit my weakness after trying so hard to be strong after Dustin's death. I had to mature to believe that natural emotions needed healthy expression rather than repression.

When someone passes away in a family, it is tempting to try to be the 'good soldier.' It's hard to show weakness, hard to admit to our pain and let someone just listen to us cry or rage. It's hard, but necessary. I hurt myself and people I cared about by repressing my emotions and letting the rage build up.

I didn't have a good answer to why God's "ways are higher than your ways." My simple and trusting childhood faith crashed hard against reality and I was left with anger and insecurity. The years after Dustin died I turned from a simple faith and tried to dull the unanswerable questions with stoicism. When my stoicism couldn't hold up against life's natural flow of emotions, often I reacted in anger or pulled away from any stimulus.

It has taken, and is still taking, a lot of effort to find balance. His thoughts are higher than my thoughts. Sometimes my thoughts have been downright chaotic and fearful. I hope God forgives me for the moments where the rage is bigger than my faith, where fear outweighs the trust, and where resentment blinds me to the love. Thank God for the chances we get to grow. We all need them.

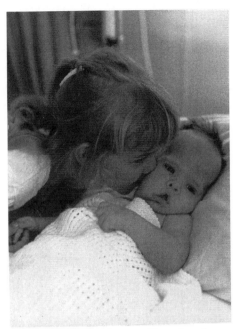

Darcy, 3, getting to know Dustin, 4 months

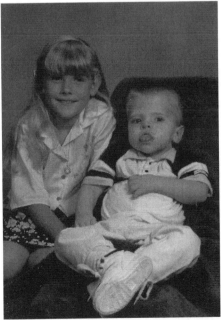

Darcy, 6, and Dustin, 3, in a family picture

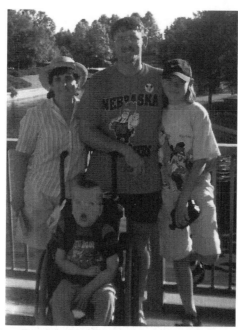

Jo Lyn, 37, Randy, 37, Darcy, 11, and Dustin 8, at Walt Disney World on Dustin's Make a Wish Trip in 1997

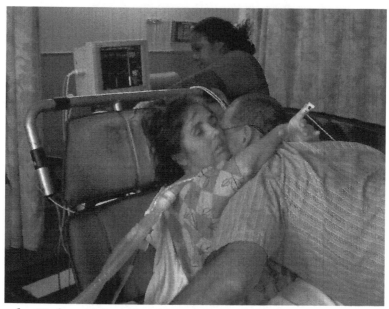

Randy, 51, hugs his wife of 30 years, Jo Lyn, 51, on a good day as she sits in her therapy chair in long term intensive care

Chapter 11
Heading Home

For the summer of 2011 Mom orchestrated a family trip to Alamogordo, New Mexico, for her grandmother's ninetieth birthday. Jo Lyn had planned a community wide celebration surprise party for my great-grandmother Grace Woolsey. The trip, and the birthday gift Mom planned for Grandma Grace, carried great importance for Mom.

At first I was reluctant to go. We had gone to New Mexico consistently for the last five or six summers, and the trips were usually around my Grandma Grace's birthday, which is three days before my husband's birthday, August 4. Spending the week with lesser-known in-laws in a small, desert city multiple years in a row didn't make Daniel feel special about his own birthday. Plus, as a married couple of teachers, it made a quick end to our summer after getting back.

Eli was going to be eight weeks old and going on a fourteen-hour car ride. Eli handled short car trips well, but longer trips were stressful. We had driven a three hour trip before with six-week-old Eli crying most the trip. I drove home the rest of the way with tight nerves after Daniel pulled over in frustration. Daniel sat in the back with closed eyes and tried to be calm as Eli screamed himself to sleep. I did not look forward to spending over twenty-four hours in a car with Eli to make the trip to New Mexico and back.

However, Mom stressed the importance of Grandma Grace's ninetieth birthday, told me how much she'd like us to come, and said the family should get the chance to meet Eli as soon as they could. We decided to drive down on our own so we could go at a slow pace for Eli so we could get home in time for him to spend his birthday with his parents and siblings.

With all the preparations that Mom had put into this trip, she wanted us to be with her for more of it, but she just thanked us for going along. We'd miss the community surprise celebration. I didn't think that was much of a loss because I wouldn't know the people there; however, my mother wanted the chance to show her former teachers and neighbors how her daughter had grown up and how cute her grandson was.

The car trip was terrible. Eli didn't like sitting in the chair longer than two hours at a time. We stopped often, sometimes twice in a town if the gas station didn't have a clean bathroom with a changing table. As inexperienced parents, we traveled with Bum Genius cloth diapers we had to keep in the back of the car and couldn't throw out. We didn't make that mistake twice though, and now travel with disposables.

We rolled into Alamagordo, my mother's hometown, at about six a.m. Daniel and I had slept in shifts, reclining in the passenger seat only when Eli was asleep and sitting next to him in the back to keep him calm while he was awake. We were frustrated, tired, and sore. Mom had spent months trying to plan a great family vacation, and I showed up exhausted and annoyed.

My great-grandmother Grace lives near the basin of a fertile mountain in a desert valley. Near the mountains there are run-off streams. It's possible, although tedious, to grow grass, and vegetation so many of the yards are rock instead. I'd lived in Mom's hometown twice: once when Dad was overseas in Korea for a year with the military building sanitation systems when I was seven and then for a year after Dad retired from the military and tried to let Mom live near her family again. We didn't have our own house either time. When I was seven, we lived with my grandma Jo Ann Talley in a two bedroom house where I had my own bedroom, my grandma had her bedroom, and Mom slept in the den on the pull-out sofa with Dustin and his equipment for almost a year. Sometimes Mom shared the bed with her mother to get a good night's sleep. She didn't have a bedroom, and most all our possessions were in storage until Dad got back and we moved back onto an Air Force base.

This vacation Daniel and I would get the bedroom with two twin beds and have Eli sleep in a travel basinet between us. My parents would again have a pull-out couch. Mom lay bundled in covers with her mouth agape and her head tilted back on two pillows. Saliva vibrated in the corner of her lip with her snoring and slowly rasping breaths. Dad lay on his side, fully clothed but with no blanket, and made eye contact as soon as we entered the door. He'd been awake already and had gone for a walk around the neighborhood.

We talked softly as most the family slept. Dad got off the bed, came over to us, and asked, "How was the drive?"

I sighed audibly, something I'd rather not have done, and brought my hand to my head to rub my forehead. "Exhausting! Eli was good when he was asleep, but we stopped more than once in the middle of nowhere so I could feed him. At least we figured out McDonalds always has changing tables. I didn't have to change him on the floor."

Dad wrapped his arms around me, putting Eli up to his chest between us, and squeezed just enough. "It really matters to your mother that you made that trip. Sorry it wasn't easy."

Daniel put the diaper bag by the wall and came to hug Dad. Daniel had woken up ten miles out of town. He yawned and said, "We took shifts driving and sleeping. I think I slept through Eli waking up a lot better than Darcy. She had to wake up every time to feed him while I drove."

I slumped into Grace's favorite chair, a large worn leather recliner I sunk into. "Are Donnie and Jessie asleep in the guest room?"

"Yeah, Don and his wife will be sleeping here. We will stay with you in the hotel."

There was empty room to nurse my son in, so I asked Daniel to unpack my nursing blanket. Stress sat on my shoulders. My body still hurt. Nursing in front of others was awkward and new.

Feeding Eli filled me with compassion. He let me caress his head as I marveled over his handsome looks and the miracle that came from my womb. Finally I was at my destination, with family, and relaxed.

"When did you guys get in?" The voice was young, timorous, the pitch of a boy nearing puberty. My cousin, Donny, had walked into the living room and stood in his pajamas with his eyes locked on my blanket and what was under it. "...Is Eli under there?"

I shifted uncomfortably, trying to ensure that nothing improper was revealed. "Yes, he's hard at work." I took a breath to calm myself. "He's eating his breakfast." I tried to smile reassuringly, but I'd never nursed around a thirteen-year-old boy.

My cousin nodded his head, his curly hair bobbing ever so slightly on his forehead. He pursed his lips, made a "hmm" sound, which sounded something like approval, smiled, and said "Cool. I'll wait to meet him." Donny headed back to his room to get dressed for family breakfast. I sighed. Breastfeeding an infant son and traveling with cloth diapers hadn't seemed ideal when we planned the trip. It was hard.

Eli finished cheerfully. I held Eli up to my face, rubbed my nose on his nose, and looked into his eyes. He smiled back at me, cooing in the language of love. We'd made it, and now my mother's family was going to meet my first born child.

As proud as I was of my son, my parents were more proud. I'm not an only child, but I am the only surviving child of a mother with a genetic disease that caused multiple miscarriages and a son who died young. My parents had been waiting, somewhat impatiently, on Eli's arrival in the world.

With the morning commotion, Mom had opened her eyes and watched me as I talked to Eli and kissed his cheek. I tickled his ribs, and a throaty push of air escaped as an infant's giggle. She smiled, and her sides moved in silent laughter along with Eli. "Carefu --" She paused to clear her throat of the gunk that had built up while she was asleep. "Careful or he'll spit up."

I turned to her. She looked so tired. The bags under her eyes were droopy and a hue of blue. Her mouth hung open, her jaw slack.

Spittle collected in the corner of her mouth. She moved her hand from under her cheek and used her arm to push herself into a sitting position, a gesture that took effort.

"He's good about keeping his milk down. I haven't been spit up on in a week or two." I stood and moved toward her. "Do you want to hold him? He's in a happy mood."

"Of course. Just let me set my feet on the floor." She positioned herself squarely on the fold-up bed, legs about shoulder-width apart. Her feet had swelled. Mom had trouble with her legs, particularly her right foot and calf. She wore a compression sock often. A fourteen hour trip was hard on her legs.

I bent over with Eli, placing him gently on her lap. I ran my thumb along the hair line of his forehead to calm him. He kept his eyes on me, so I smiled to comfort him. "You be a good boy for Grandma. She loves you and wants to show you off today to her family."

Mom snuggled Eli to her chest. He rested his head in the soft skin near her elbow, content in arms that had already held him so many times. Mom was genuinely happy. She leaned in close and spoke soft words, her eyes alert and lively. I thought about the two of them together. Summer was coming to an end, and she was supposed to come spend the next few months living with Daniel and me in the guest bedroom as a live-in babysitter. She had grown frustrated and lonely in Larned. Taking care of Eli seemed like worthwhile work. It was our chance to reconnect.

I was important to Mom, and living away from me had been increasingly difficult for her. In the month before the trip to New Mexico, Mom had become nearly impossible to understand on the phone. I'd let her talk but didn't catch much. I didn't want to ask "What?" ten times because I knew it would frustrate her and she couldn't fix the problem. She'd realize I didn't know what she was saying or think I wasn't paying attention when I'd say "yeah" to the wrong thing. She'd get frustrated, both at herself and at me. Then the phone conversation would end soon after. Our phone conversations went from thirty minutes to three. Then Mom wouldn't call every day. Sometimes, she wouldn't answer when I called. I was glad to be with her in person. Watching her hold Eli, I felt hope. Mom could live with me, be happy with Eli, and we could talk again.

After a failed phone call with Mom a week earlier, I cried to my husband and said, "I feel like I'm losing my mother."

We knew her health was getting worse. Daniel and I discussed the risks of letting her take care of Eli. Originally, she was going to stay with us until summer. Then, she said she would do it until Christmas break. We planned to have a stroller in the house she could use to move Eli from room to room. I wanted my healthy son to bring new hope for my ailing mother.

"Breakfast is ready," Grace called from the kitchen, her ninety-year-old voice shaky. "Come to the table, and we'll pray."

Mom lifted Eli for me to grab. She set her feet squarely on the ground, put both arms on the edge of the bed and pushed. Her lips rose, and her teeth showed, but she didn't get up from that sunk-in sleeper bed. She reached out a hand. "Help me up?"

I shifted Eli and pulled her with my free hand. She grabbed my hand with her right hand then clasped her left hand on top. She came to her feet with a good pull from me. "Thank you, thank you," she said, in good spirits, smiling bigger than she had to.

She had slept in her clothes from driving. As she walked, the pants leg over her compression sock stuck above her calf. Her steps were small, and she teetered slightly from side to side. After about six steps she stumbled slightly but caught her hand on the wall and moved on as if nothing had happened. Two steps later she was holding onto her chair at the table, steady and balanced.

Breakfast felt good. Eli was fed and happy, my cousins were excited to see us, Great-grandmother Grace had energy, and Mom basked in the accomplishment of her goal of getting her family together to celebrate Grace's birthday. It seemed the trip would go well, even if I already dreaded the drive back to Kansas. I caught a nap with Eli after lunch, and that evening we made our way to White Sands National Park as we do every time we visit New Mexico.

White Sands was a family tradition. Monochrome color pictures with white borders and beveled edges from the 1970s showed my mom at White Sands as a skinny attractive young woman who fit in with everyone else her age. My uncle Don had grown up playing Frisbee on the tops of the dunes. Mom had made the same grade school field trip I did. Daniel had sealed a friendship with my cousin Tanya's husband, Jeremiah, by letting Jeremiah push him down the well-grooved track with the sand ramp at the bottom. Daniel flew off the plastic saucer used in Kansas for snow and in New Mexico on desert dunes, landed on his shoulder, and rolled gracefully into a full-bellied laugh. My family had been out there on every trip we took to New Mexico, sometimes more than once. The last National Park that Dustin visited was White Sands in 2001.

Dustin had loved White Sands. How does a boy in a wheelchair come to love a park that requires lots of walking and climbing and has no air conditioning past the gift shop? Piggy back rides from Dad, a sand shovel, and a pail he could fill and dump. Dustin would sit in one spot, usually shaded by a larger dune, and enjoy the gypsum sand running through his fingers, filling his shovel, and pouring out of his pail, usually onto some part of his body.

My fondest memory of White Sands was Dustin's last trip. I was sixteen and loved the outdoors and physical challenge. I ran hard along the hills until dusk. Normally, when the sun went down we'd leave. There aren't street lights along the dunes, and fires are prohibited. However, this night, Dustin's last night at the dunes, there was a meteor storm that was supposed to be visible in the night sky. White Sands was the best place to see it. My family had laid out blankets on the top of a dune. After running ragged, I sat there and sifted gypsum through my fingers with Dustin. We played together on that dune, Dad, Dustin, and me, all sitting in one spot and waiting for the meteor shower to appear. Mom sat contently with her sister, Donna, her niece, Tanya, and her mother, Jo Ann. We talked, we laughed, and we listened. Life slowed down, waiting for a 'shooting star' to cross the sky while we enjoyed nature's splendor and majesty in a place entrenched in my family's history.

As I lay on my back, blanket under me and fingers wrapped behind my head, one streak of light flashed across the sky, then another, followed by more in a stream of space rubble burning in the atmosphere. In the middle of a desert in a landscape so desolate that our government chose the deeper dune area for atomic bomb testing, that night I felt the magnitude of life. I had enough independence and physical blessings to challenge myself to run the dunes, and I had the security and comfort of family to ground me in my roots, a brother to remind me of the simple joys in life, and Mom to support me in whatever I chose to do. I thought that night fortuitous then, a sign to count my blessings and enjoy what was.

That summer, at eight weeks old, Eli took his first visit to the dunes. We drove out in a caravan of cars, Daniel and I riding with Eli; Dad drove Mom, Grandma Jo, and Grandma Grace; Tanya brought Jeremiah and their two daughters, Sophie and Ellie; and my uncle Don and his wife Julie brought Donny and Jessica. We paid our way and drove through the flatter section of the park, where yucca plants could be seen pushing through the gypsum and man-made bridges had been laid out in parks for guided tours. Eventually the two-lane road was compacted with gypsum at the edge of either side of the pavement. We kept driving until the two lanes became one because the gypsum covered the outer two feet on each side of the asphalt where the tire tracks were not as fresh.

I pried Eli from the car seat and carried him over to the covered picnic table, hiding from the sun on a ninety-degree day in the New Mexico desert. He slept. Mom brought over her sandwich fixings and sat next to us, making a sandwich for me first.

"He looks so restful in your arms." She put her fingers on my arm that held Eli and leaned in to peer at his face. I crossed my other hand over Eli and covered Mom's hand with my own. A proud smile crossed my lips.

"He likes to sleep during car trips." I paused, remembering Eli's cries on the fourteen-hour trip to New Mexico. "Short car trips, anyway."

Mom laughed almost inaudibly, the air coming mostly out her nose. "Car trips aren't as easy as they used to be, are they? I slept most the trip. My body is so sore. It's hard to elevate my leg in the car for that long. I'm glad White Sands is a short trip."

I leaned my head onto her shoulder, resting on her cushion-like flesh. "I'm tired, Momma. I've haven't gotten eight hours of sleep since my second trimester. In the car I got to sleep a little but woke up every time Eli cried so we could pull over and change his diaper or feed him." Daniel had gotten a circular snow sled saucer from Tanya and was running up the dune. "I just want to sit here with you."

We sat and ate slowly, talked about motherhood, relaxed as others struggled against the sand in a pilgrimage to the top of the dune, and took turns holding Eli. I slowed my pace, enjoying the fun of others as I rested with Mom.

Daniel, with sand in his sweaty hair came over with a request. "Come with me. I've got a great path all smooth so you'll go fast." He held his saucer in one hand, the other moving toward the bread.

I reached out to grab the bread before he did. "How about you sit down and I'll make you a sandwich." He sat, talked a little to Mom, and ate the sandwich quickly. He was eager for the fun of the dunes again.

"I want to take Eli down the dune."

"What?" I asked incredulously.

"I want to hold him as I go down on the saucer."

"He's eight weeks old. Why does he need to go down a dune?"

"It's tradition. Why not? He only gets the chance when we are here."

I looked down at my son, who was now awake. He was content, quietly taking in his surroundings. "He's tired."

"He's on vacation. He doesn't need to just sit around." And with that, Daniel was off with one hand holding the saucer and one arm carrying his son.

I looked at Mom, who, from her seat, pointed her finger and called at Daniel's back "You better not hurt him. Be careful!"

Daniel replied, "I will. Grab a camera; I want a picture."

I complied, getting the camera out of the diaper bag. My spirit was conflicted. Daniel was young and active, and as someone whose body was still recovering from bearing a child, I felt more like my mother, wanting to just sit and observe. Part of me wanted to go slide the dunes with Daniel, part of me wanted to run after him and take back my son, and another part of me just wanted to sit there and hold my breath.

I sat and held my breath, camera in hand. Daniel reached the top of the dune, positioned the saucer in the middle of the smooth track, sat cross legged in the middle, and sat Eli in his lap between his legs. He wrapped one arm around Eli and used the other arm to push against the sand and start the saucer down the dune. The saucer slid down the dune, picking up speed as it went. The saucer twisted, and Daniel's feet were no longer in front. He was approaching the small ramp at the bottom with my son in his arms, and he couldn't see where he was going. My chest tightened, and my throat seemed to rise toward my mouth. Daniel put out his arm to drag in the sand and right his direction. He approached the ramp, still backwards. He shot out one leg, dragging it in the sand too, then rolled off the saucer onto the side of the path, cradling Eli is his right arm as he again found his feet. It could be called graceful and athletic, or stupid. Regardless of what I could call it, Eli was safe, still content.

Mom did not enjoy the scene. When Daniel began to roll, Mom tried to get up from the picnic table. She put her arms down on the table and tried to push herself up and sideways to get out. From the corner of my eye, I saw her grimace and move about six inches. In that same time, Daniel had completed his role, checked Eli, and stood on his feet. Mom wanted to run to her grandson, but she was too slow, too weak. She did get off the picnic bench on her own, but by that time Daniel was walking back towards us with a dumb-luck adventurer's grin across his face.

Mom sat the rest of the night in a fold-up chair in the shade of the picnic awning. For a while we kept talking and made sure Eli didn't have hidden battle wounds. Soon enough though, I ran off after a saucer and up a dune with Daniel, leaving Mom content with Eli.

Mom would have loved for me to stay longer to chat. As her only living child, I was her pride and joy. However, as she aged and the muscle weakness progressed, she sometimes observed more than she interacted. Often, she walked behind the group unless someone was conscientious enough to walk beside her. When we went to active places, she usually sat near the car or entrance and watched. When I was near her, I often engaged in activity she wasn't physically ready to endure rather than being near her for conversation. I would slow down for my ninety-year-old great-grandmother or my infant son. I suppose I still thought of Mom as the physically capable woman who chased me down the hall when I was six or coached my t-ball team when I was four.

Mom had a disease creeping inside her muscles, degenerating her muscle strength even in the supposedly safe confines of her own bed or kitchen. I could have been more considerate, and engaged her in conversation rather than left her with my baby and run off to do something I'd done a hundred times before. I acted normally, which is to say blindly. With Dustin, we knew to value him as if each day were his last. With Mom, her weakness approached infinitesimally more each day. Instead of understanding and cherishing my moments with her, I took for granted that she should act like she had before, and that when she looked well, she felt well. There was so much I missed.

I value the moments I listened to Mom, where I slowed down because I was tired. Mom's pace may have seemed tired judging from the outside, but it was her pace, appropriate to what she was feeling on the inside. Slowing down to listen or show someone they are valued is a beautiful gesture of love and compassion. Slowing down for too long seems un-American; it's not progressive. We are so adventure driven, goal oriented, or entertainment based. I wish I had spent more time at Mom's pace. I often looked past the value of those moments, even when I knew what I should do. I could have sat more often with Mom to do a puzzle, watch a soap opera, or look through her quilting material. I took those small moments for granted, in part because day to day I couldn't see a change in my mother. She was weakening, changing, and unfortunately, I wasn't aware or wise enough to change with her and embrace the time I had with her.

After running the dunes, playing Frisbee on the flats, and burying my younger cousins in sand, I eventually returned to Mom. She sat slumped in the chair, holding Eli against her shoulder as he gummed her clavicle. She looked up at me. Her eyes were tired, red, glossy; I thought her allergies were agitated. She smiled as best she could. I thought I had hurt her feelings when I left her holding Eli and run off. Her smile was lopsided. One end of her lips curled up more than the other.

"He's hungry. He's been trying to eat my shoulder for a few minutes now." Her voice was kind. I didn't detect any resentment.

"I'll take him. Just give me a minute." Eli moved his head at my voice, crying in hunger. I attempted to knock the sand off, washed my hands with a water bottle, and got my nursing cover from the car. I pulled the green fold-up travel chair closer to Mom and took my mewing son.

We talked -- about what I did at the dunes, advice about Eli, Mom's church in Larned, Grace's upcoming birthday. The topics weren't the point; we were both just glad to sit and talk successfully. That was all that mattered. I spent the last twenty minutes of our four-hour trip to White Sands talking with Mom.

That night the five of us slept in a two-queen-bed hotel room. Daniel and I shared a bed with Eli in a travel basinet on the floor. Daniel did not wake when Eli cried or squirmed. I, however, woke every time Eli cried, changed his diaper, and fed him. I didn't get much sleep. Mom snored lightly as she slept. I woke up grumpy and tired.

Mom woke up slowly and still groggy. Her legs were puffiest in the mornings. She sat on the edge of her bed with unfocused eyes, her mouth agape. She looked dazed. I told her good morning, to which she nodded and said something indistinguishable like 'mornin.' I had watched her put the compression sleeve on her leg before, but not in the morning during the last few months.

First, she put large yellow rubber gloves on both hands. Then, she grabbed the skin-colored nylon mesh-looking leg sleeve from the nightstand and, while sitting on the bed, tried to lift her leg into the opening of the sleeve. She nearly fell over. She huffed in frustration and rebalanced herself. She tried again, bending over further in an attempt to not have to raise her foot far. The bed in the hotel was taller than the one at her home. That didn't work either.

"Darcy, can you get your father?" Her eyes drooped. "I can't do this without him." The skin under her eyes had a blue tint. Her lips were loose and seemed to have a natural frown. I got Dad. He helped Mom do something that most days she could do independently. We went to eat lunch with family then drove up the mountain to the Ruidoso Downs Race Track. Mom sat in her seat at the horse races and didn't leave it until it started to rain on us after two hours. Mom seemed happy to be surrounded by her family, though maybe hot and slightly uncomfortable. She did complain once, about the heat making her light-headed.

That night, after we returned, we all dressed for a big family dinner and gathered to take pictures. A hand-stitched floral décor cooking apron hung over Grandma Jo Ann's neck as she hunted for her camera. "Darcy, I want a picture of you, your son, and Daniel first. Stand over there by the white wall."

Obliging, we stood there by the wall and waited patiently as three different people tried to get Eli to look at the camera long enough to get a family photo. My cheeks were sore by the time Eli cooperated. Grandma Jo called another command. "Mom, you get in this picture too. We need a picture of you and Eli."

Great-grandmother Grace hobbled out of her chair, gingerly grabbed her walker with both hands, and pushed her way to where we stood. She left the walker by the wall just out of range of the picture and began walking towards me.

Grandma Jo's voice raised in concern. "Mother, you know you can't walk without your walker. You need that!"

"Oh, I'll just stand here for a picture. I'll be fine." Grace grabbed my waist and held on next to me, smiling.

Grandma Jo raised her camera, saying as she took the picture, "You fell just last week. The doctor told you not to walk anywhere without it anymore. You're going to have to get used to that." She moved the camera down and looked her mother in the eyes. "Okay?"

"Okay, I will. Just take the picture, dear. Eli is so cute." Grace looked at Eli and smiled. She whispered to me, "He looks just like you and your mom did as babies." We smiled genuinely together.

"Now I want a five generation photo." Jo Ann was excited. "Here, Daniel. You take the picture. Jo Lyn, come over here and take a picture with us."

Mom was sitting at the couch, comfortably observing. She leaned, put her weight on her arm, and tried to heave herself out of the couch. It took two attempts. She shuffled in little steps toward where we were standing. Her leg rubbed on the coffee table between her and us, and she stumbled but caught herself and kept walking. She was still slightly off balance and took three more steps before bumping into me. I stepped back to keep my balance, which was difficult with Eli in tow. My hip bumped Grace, who let out a gentle "oh."

Mom grabbed the shoulder of my arm holding Eli and used me to rebalance. My spine bent backwards. I grunted and pulled myself forward. I grabbed her with my free arm and held her steady.

"Sorry, didn't mean to do all that." She smiled at me, opening her mouth a bit to show her teeth in an obvious attempt to please me. I let out my breath in frustration.

I blurted "Mom, how are you going to take care of Eli this fall if you can't even walk without stumbling?" Her feeble smile disappeared. Her tears welled before I finished the sentence.

"I don't know!" Mom stammered, something between a yell and a cry.

There was an awkward silence. I squeezed her arm, trying with a physical gesture to say sorry. She wouldn't look at me. She wiped the tears away with her thumb quickly, hoping no one noticed. She looked at Daniel, who was holding the camera, and attempted to smile. Daniel looked at me with questions in his eyes. I nodded my head as a signal to go on.

"Alright, everyone smile," Daniel said.

Dad called for Eli's attention with odd noises and funny faces. We all smiled, or rather, tried. Mom could not get a smile across her face.

"Jo Lyn, that's not a smile," Grandma Jo called to her. "That doesn't even lift your cheeks, much less get to your eyes." Jo Ann, the mother, smiled at Jo Lyn, her daughter, as if she were giving an example to a reticent eight-year-old, showing extra teeth and big eyes.

Mom tried; she honestly did. Her bottom lip dropped further down, but her upper lip didn't rise. Her body failed her. Her expression looked more like a snarl than a smile.

"Smile big, like this." Grace showed a full toothy grin to Mom, who tried to appear happy. Mom's cheeks sagged, and her whole appearance seemed loose, sad, fatigued. Anxiety consumed her face.

She turned toward the camera one more time and tried to raise her lips.

"Are you smiling?" Daniel asked, wondering if he should take the picture.

Mom threw her hands in the air. "I can't!" She wailed. "I can't smile right now!" With that she left, ambling off toward the bathroom.

I regretted what I said before all the words had left my mouth. I had made Mom cry on a trip she'd looked forward to for a year. Yet my regret mixed with a protective feeling. Something said, 'This must be done for the safety of my child.' Daniel and I wondered whether Mom would be able to care for Eli without accidently harming him. Daniel had pulled me aside earlier that day to discuss his concerns about Mom's endurance and balance.

"We have to tell her we need to find someone else. She'll drop him. It isn't safe."

His words haunted me. She wasn't physically capable of carrying Eli safely with no one else home. I wanted her to watch Eli, though. I wanted her to share that joy with me. Her self-worth was gratified even when I just asked her questions about motherhood. She felt needed, necessary -- she had a purpose.

That day, posing for a picture, I reacted with pent-up emotion of losing an opportunity I yearned for. I didn't react with sympathy, I didn't take time to think, and I didn't ask if she were okay. I just tried to protect my son. In the process I hurt my mother.

Dad told me later that she cried in the bathroom then cried when he took her to the bedroom. She wanted to take care of Eli as much as, if not more than, I wanted her to. Mom felt small, as if she were a nuisance, a danger to her grandson. I can only guess what else she felt, what she knew about her own body, what she thought of her own future.

The next day was Grace's birthday and the last full day Daniel and I planned to stay in New Mexico. At dinner that night we had all the family in town together and crowded around Grace's table. After we cleaned up, Mom sat smiling at her place at the dinner table, her fingers neatly crossed in front of her and some light to her eyes. She asked Dad, "Randy, can you go get the gift?"

He came back with a blue-covered scrapbook that had hand-placed sticker wording on the front. Grace smiled as it was set in front of her, her wrinkles lifting up into dimples. Her grateful eyes and her soft, worn hand traced the edge of the scrapbook before opening it. "My, what is this? It looks like you spent so much time doing it." She ran her fingers along the letters, photographs, and decorations.

Mom's chest rose in pride. Her chin rested on her hand, and she leaned forward to share with her grandmother: "This is a picture of you and granddad that I got from Aunt Leora. Do you remember that?"

Grace looked at the picture for a long time and pursed her lips together, enjoying the memory. "Why, yes I do. That is Don at one of his first jobs after I married him. He's working for the Works Progress Administration during the Depression." She looked up at Mom and smiled until her cheeks lifted her glasses. "We didn't have much, but he worked so hard. He left me a nice house and steady life. He was a good man."

Softly, Mom laughed. "You like it, do you?" she asked tenderly, having put hours of work into cutting and gluing.

"Oh, yes. This is the best birthday gift I've gotten in a long time. It means so much to me to have my memories right here in front of me. You sure outdid yourself." Grace delighted in flipping through the pictures. "Where did you get this picture of Bobby? I don't think I've ever seen it."

Mom leaned affectionately closer to her grandmother. "That's the trailer he shared with Amy. It came from my collection. I kept every picture I had of Bobby when he passed away. They are in with the same box as Dustin's." Her eyes stayed even; her face didn't drop. Her brother, Robert "Bobby" Woodard, passed away at age thirty one from a moped accident shortly before Dustin passed. Bobby likely had undiagnosed myotonic muscular dystrophy inherited from their father. In school he was labeled with a broad learning disability. He and Mom were close. Sometimes the mention of his name made Mom sad.

No tears welled in her eyes. She was happy, proud to share her year's hard work with her aging grandmother. They glowed over the book for almost an hour together before it got passed around to other family members. When I got my chance to look, Grace peered over my shoulder occasionally, and Mom actively answered questions about my relatives.

I hope when I turn ninety I get a gift like that for my birthday and get to spend hours basking with my descendants over the beautiful days gone by and fondly remember those who are no longer here. I'd be blessed one day to have a granddaughter, like Mom was to Grace, who would plan a present for me for a whole year, contact family members for resources, hand-lay the pages, and drive across five states to give it to me. Jo Lyn's best talent in life was to make those close to her feel exceptionally loved. She was devotedly loyal, supportive regardless of the doubts, and thought constantly about how to make the lives of those she loved just a little bit better. Some of the words had off-center letters or were misspelled. Some of the pictures had ink lines or crooked lines in the cutting. It didn't matter. So much grateful love went into making the book that Mom's faithful character overtook her decreasing manual dexterity and created a true symbol of love.

Mom was happy that day. She sat on the couch and held Eli while he slept. I rested with my head on her lap as she stroked my hair. We went over and over her scrapbook and the stories of her making it. Her grandmother was grateful, her mother was proud, and I was inspired.

While we were all chatting, Mom mentioned at various times feeling light-headed and dizzy and having odd dreams. She didn't sleep well, and at the hotel she actually slept with three pillows propped behind her back, practically sitting her up. Dad and I talked and thought it might be allergies in the area or elevation sickness from going up the mountains to the horse races the day prior. Mom mentioned her symptoms one at a time in separate conversations. She didn't want to make it the central issue of the day.

Grandma Jo saw the good mood of everyone around the living room and wanted a second shot at pictures. Uncle Don's family took pictures, Tanya's family took pictures, Mom's sister Donna took pictures with her girls, Daniel and I took pictures with Eli, and then Mom and Dad took pictures, all on Grace's back porch in her gliding bench.

My parents rarely both smiled in a picture. They stood there, arms wrapped around each other, with the kind of smiles that come from a couple married for over twenty years who only take pictures when other people ask them to.

We lined up to try our five generation photo again. Holding my sleeping son, I sat on the bench next to Grace. Jo Ann went behind the bench, as did my mother. Grandma Jo put Mom's arm between hers to give Mom extra stability. We looked toward three different photographers, all saying, 'Smile' or 'Look here.'

Grandma Jo looked over at Mom and asked, "Jo Lyn, are you trying to smile?"

Mom's cheeks tightened. "Yes, I am. Does it not look like it?"

"Maybe you should try to open your eyes more or lift your eyebrows."

One of the pictures I have from that day has Mom with big eyes, lifted eyebrows, and a flat upper lip. There is no curve to her smile. Her lower lip hangs open with a droopy expression. Something was wrong with Mom if she couldn't smile, as happy as she was. I thought once we got her home to Kansas she would recover. It had to be the mountain climate, allergens from a state she didn't live in, not sleeping well in a hotel, or the consequences of spending fourteen hours in a car.

We spent the rest of the night enjoying family. Later, Mom asked if I could stay longer and go to the community birthday party for Grace. "It's been so good having you here, Darcy. Can you stay one more day?"

"Mom, I've really enjoyed being here, but it's hard on me and Eli. I want to go back to my own bed. I've been tired all week. Plus, Daniel hasn't been home for his birthday for two years. I need to make that happen for him. We are leaving tomorrow like we planned."

"I know. I'm just really going to miss you. It isn't the same when you aren't around. You and Eli are such a blessing." She hugged my arm and rested her soft, floppy cheek on my shoulder. "You don't come to visit me very often anymore."

I sighed. Feeling guilty agitated me. "It's just harder to drive down that highway since we hit the deer at night. There are so many deer between Salina and Larned. I don't like to drive that way at night anymore." I looked at her to meet her eyes. "I'll bring Eli by more when he handles car rides better. And soon you'll be living with us and taking care of him when school starts. We'll see lots of each other soon, Mom."

"When does school start for you again?"

"In about two weeks. Are you packed and ready? I have the guest room ready for you."

She hesitated. "I don't know." Her eyes looked hollow, a bottomless blue, a shade of pain, a color of fear. "I'll get ready."

"We have a stroller that fits all the doorways. We'll keep it in Eli's room near his crib so he'll be easier to move from room to room."

She turned her eyes from me and rested her head on my shoulder again. "That'll help. I worry about carrying him all over. I get tired."

I hugged my mother. "We'll make it work, Mom. You're going to help me learn to be as good of a mother to Eli as you were to me. I'm excited."

She hugged me as her face sunk into my chest. "I love you. You mean so much to me. Thank you for giving me a grandson. He's very handsome."

"He is cute. There are many things I don't know, Mom. Having a baby in the house is a lot to handle. I'm glad I'll have you around in the next couple months."

"Yeah, those will be good times." She sat up and wiped her eyes. "Let's go enjoy the rest of the night while you're here."

"Okay, Mom. I bet we can wait until after lunch to leave tomorrow. That'll give us one more family dinner."

We stayed the next day until after lunch. Then we left for home.

That was the last time I would see my mother outside of a hospital.

Chapter 12
The Smell of Clean

When Dustin died, a part of what formed my character was no longer visible to the outside world. Somehow, without a blatant visual reminder of the genetic disease in my family, I almost forgot it was there. I didn't have any more the regular trips to the hospital where doctors would coach me on how to help my affected family members. I thought Mom was suffering from allergies or would recover normally. She was getting weaker, but I didn't recommend we take her to a doctor right away. She didn't have folders upon folders of medical records like Dustin. I didn't look after my mother in the same way I did my brother. I was more worried about my son than Mom. I was caught off guard the day I got the call.

My phone rang in the kitchen while Daniel and I were visiting with his mother at our home in Salina. I went to the back porch to answer it while Daniel and his mom continued an in-depth conversation.

"Hi, Darcy. I love you very, very much." Dad's voice was extra cheery, and an opener like that let me know there was trouble. It was August 5, the day after my husband's birthday and my parents' first day back in Kansas.

"Hey, Dad. What's up?" I asked.

"Well, I'm going to take your mother to the hospital. She hasn't been staying awake or alert since we left New Mexico. I'm sure they can give her something to clear her up." He still explained in his cheery hopeful voice.

"I can get Eli in the car and leave in about 10 minutes --" I was going to say more.

"No. Don't do that. I'm not sure whether they'll have to keep her or just give her a breathing treatment or something. I'll call when I know more."

I sat on the porch stairs for a few minutes. Fear sank in. Small signs in New Mexico pointed to a larger issue. I wondered what could "clear up" Mom -- if they had something to clear all the allergens from her system or some type of altitude detox for people coming back from mountains to the prairie. I wasn't hopeful. If it were her MMD...

I went back inside and sat and listened to a conversation that was intensifying rather than winding down. My mother-in-law looked near tears, and my husband was trying to be tender. It seemed like an important moment for mother and son, so I waited. I waited on that phone call and didn't tell Daniel my mother was going to the hospital. I waited and let Eli sleep longer.

The second phone call came about ten minutes later.

"They don't have facilities for her here in Larned. The breathing treatment didn't fix things. She's taking another nebulizer."

"Okay. Daniel and Carolyn are talking, but we could leave." I hesitated, uncertain of what to do. "Should we come down?"

"No. The ambulance isn't in town. They had to call the ambulance back in from another out-of-town run. It might be awhile before we go anywhere. I'll call you when we get there."

This time I sat on the back porch and cried. Waiting felt terrible.

The third time the phone rang was a good deal of time later and not my father.

"Hi, Darcy. Have you heard your mother is in the hospital?" It was my Uncle Michael.

"Yeah. Dad called and told me the ambulance was going to take her to Hays. Have you seen her?"

"No. We are at Hays, though. Are you going to come stay the night? If you aren't, let me know; I'll take the day off and stay here." His voice was businesslike. I almost felt he was disappointed in me for not already being on the road.

"Stay the night? My dad said it wasn't serious and should clear up."

"He's going to need someone here. Can you come down?" I knew from his tone then that Dad had been protecting me. That too-cheery voice couldn't bear to tell me how scared he was. Dad thought it was his job all those years with Dustin to be the rock of the family. He didn't have it in him to ask me to come down to be his emotional support. Dad wouldn't tell me that Mom's condition was serious with a grim outlook. His brother's voice did, though.

I walked back in the door ready to alarm my family. "Daniel, my mother is being taken by ambulance to Hays Medical Center."

"What? That's terrible! We should leave now." He knew what the news meant after seeing Mom in New Mexico.

I looked down at the carpet and played with my fingers. "She isn't there yet. The ambulance had to drive from somewhere else to pick her up. We can wait if you and your mother still need to talk."

Carolyn answered for herself. "No, I'll be fine. Daniel has been very supportive, and I feel like I can get through this. You go be with your mother."

We packed up Eli and drove over the speed limit to Hays, a town of about 20,000 in Western Kansas.

By the time we arrived at the hospital in Hays, Mom was non-responsive. She was tired and drugged past the point of holding conversation. The doctor in the Intensive Care Unit (ICU) wanted to intubate her — put a tube down her throat so that a machine could help her breathe. My parents had previously discussed their will, what would happen if either died, their final requests for burial, and whether or not life support should be used. Jo Lyn and Randy had told each other that they didn't want to live on life support, but Mom did not carry a 'do not resuscitate' card in her wallet. Since she couldn't answer for herself and Dad wasn't sure what she'd want in this situation, Dad told the doctor to wait at least a day to try to see if Mom could answer herself.

She had seemed healthy enough the week before, not dying. There was no catastrophic accident, and it seemed reasonable that a lung infection had caused the condition more than a terminal illness because the change happened so quickly. Letting her die slowly due to carbon dioxide shutting down her body rather than using the assistance of a machine to support her breathing felt premature. Mom's health had been slowly declining for years. This felt like falling off a cliff. Jo Lyn's myotonic muscular dystrophy couldn't have progressed so quickly that one day she could host a party for her grandma Grace and two days later be in the ICU, taking her last natural breaths. Surely the quick decline had to be a virus. Surely the pneumonia could be fought off; she could regain strength and continue to live at home for at least a few more years.

Randy, Eli, and I stayed that night in a hotel while Mom rested in the hospital hooked to an IV, heavily sedated, unable to speak and seemingly unconscious. My father and son cuddled that night until Eli fell asleep, and then I moved Eli to his portable crib. Dad wept quietly, scared of the impending decision that he had delayed. Perhaps I should have left Eli in his arms.

Dad woke early and left to go try to talk to his ailing wife while Eli and I still slept. The exhaustion that set in that morning was deeper than the physical sleep deprivation that is the standard with a new child. It was the exhaustion of mental stress, a broken heart, and an uncertain future for the most important woman in my life. I left New Mexico knowing Mom wasn't healthy. I didn't expect our last full conversation with real words and healthy bodies to be my telling Mom I was headed home and her asking me to stay longer. Had she thought that might be the last time she saw me?

I slept with the exhaustion of regret, woke in the middle of the night, and couldn't go back to sleep with the weariness of uncertainty. I lay in my hotel bed in Hays, Kansas, August 17, 2011, five feet from Eli in his portable bed, isolated from the power to change my fate and lonely from missing the vivacious, healthy, happy mother I once had. What was in Mom's future? Did she have a future? Awake with a racing mind, I gathered Eli in my arms and wept silently, my chin resting on the top of his head.

Daniel had come down with us the first day but returned home with the car that night to go teach on the first day of school in the morning. I was still on maternity leave. I waited, cried and prayed in that hotel alone with Eli.

When Dad returned, he warned me about what to expect: Mom was weak, for the most part stuck in bed, and hadn't made it to the bathroom last time she tried. However, she was responsive in a way that allowed her to smile, nod, and understand simple questions. She wasn't able to speak. Some level of communication would be possible, but Mom was weakened and drugged. Eli would not be allowed near her due to his young immune system and the harmful germs present in any ICU. Mom had a respiratory infection— likely pneumonia.

Dad drove us to the hospital, mostly in silence, with only a few short phrases spoken between father and daughter. We had family that had come to Hays and offered to watch Eli in the waiting room so Dad and I could go in together.

Dad smiled and said, "C'mon, kiddo." He offered his hand and pulled me from my seat. His bulky fingers comfortably dwarfed my own. It was as if I were little again and he were leading me on a trip to see Dustin, ready to explain the world and the nature of sickness and weakness after we all got to go home together. Sickness seemed safer when I was young. That morning, I had heard Dad weep on his pillow.

We walked hand in hand down a well-lit, long hallway. Our footsteps echoed in unison off the clean, white walls. Dad's grip tightened, and I could feel his pulse against my fingers. I squeezed back, stealing a glance at his face, noticing the shallow features of his neck, the veins standing out against his skin, the gaunt tightness of his chin, and the clamp of his teeth. I rarely saw him nervous. The echo of my heels reverberated in my ears. I imagined I could hear the desperate pulsing of my father's heart. It was probably my own.

In every memory I have I knew Dustin would die before me. I assumed the same thing about my parents. Dad walked the halls to his weakened wife, who gave birth to a congenitally and terminally ill son and carried a hidden disease that may have been failing her lungs at that very moment. No one had told him when he was younger that he would outlive his child and wife. No one had raised him to think he was built to survive the deaths from unhealthy genetics in the family. Dad hadn't been raised for this day. If I were to describe fear as a smell in my life, it would radiate of the daily cleaning supplies of hospitals. The place reeked of fear; it overwhelmed me.

We walked through two hallways and a doorway to reach the ICU from the waiting room. We walked silently as the click of our feet reverberated off those overly clean walls. The light cream walls, the white tile with little whimsy or decoration, those strong overhead lights – everything was white, bright, and clean. Dad pushed open the door to the ICU. The desk nurse looked up. It was early enough in the morning that she smiled. "Are you here to see your wife?"

"Yes, and this is our daughter, Darcy."

I nodded, quickly and awkwardly, as my stomach dropped to my feet. Raised with a brother so often in the hospital, waiting rooms were fine, safe. An ICU, however, meant something serious. The thicker the scent of cleaner is in the hospital, the more serious the illness.

"Can you please use the hand sanitizer by the door before entering? Your mother napped after your father left. She's still rather drowsy."

I squirted the cold gel of the hand sanitizer in my hand. The scent prickled my nostril. This was real; crisis was inescapable. This was no waiting room, no regular checkup. I spread the liquid over my hands. Goosebumps pricked up on my arms and a chill ran down my spine.

Dad and I walked to the last room on the left. Every room we passed had more machines than people. The door to Mom's room was wide open. She was lying on her back, with the hospital bed inclined so that her head rested on a pillow with her chin tilted towards the air, her open mouth agape. Her lips were like the New Mexico landscape we left behind, dry and cracked. Mom didn't look peaceful. Resting didn't look restful.

Dad's voice was boisterous, yearning for hope in the too clean, too bright ICU by being too loud. "Hey, Jo Lyn, your daughter is here to see you. Wake up and smile for her."

Mom stirred just enough to indicate visibly that she registered something around her. Her eyes fluttered, her machines beeped, and still she lay. She had wires taped to her fingers, a needle stuck in her arm, three different screen monitors in the room, and no open eyes to greet me with. I gave Dad a tight lipped half smile, signaling it was okay to leave her to rest.

I drifted toward the monitor with green lights. Her first number was not green. Her oxygenation number was in the lower 80s. Not green meant not good. Dad said she was dizzy, light-headed, and had slept constantly on the way home from New Mexico. She was sleeping in a near comatose state when he came home for lunch and took her to the ER in Larned.

Her brain was not getting enough oxygen, and that was why they wanted to put tubes in her throat, to fill her lungs and supply her brain. Her pulse rate was green, which was good enough, but I had no idea what type of medication was in her body to try to retain that equilibrium.

Low oxygenation meant sleepiness and general unresponsiveness. I didn't expect her to converse with me anytime soon. In a quiet voice, I told my father, "Dad, I think she needs her rest."

"She was just talking to me before I left to pick you up from the hotel. She can talk to you now, but if we intubate her, she won't be able to talk with the tubes in." The blacks of his eyes were tighter, blacker. His gaze was earnest, frantic. He wanted me to be able to speak with Mom now - because I might never get the chance again.

I went over to her and wrapped my fingers around hers, noticing the needle marks on her fingers and arms. I held her hand, moved my face towards hers, told her I loved her in the voice I use to put Eli to sleep, and kissed her gently on the cheek. I held my face near hers and listened for breath - raspy, slow, weak. There was a tube that is worn around the face and puts oxygen into a patient's nostrils hanging on one of the monitors.

I pointed to the oxygen tube and asked, "Why isn't she wearing that?"

"Her numbers were good this morning," Dad said hopefully. "They want to see how well she breathes on her own."

I glanced again at the yellow number on the monitor. "It doesn't look like she's getting enough oxygen on her own. If we want to talk to her, maybe she should wear that for a while. Maybe she'll have enough energy to wake up then."

Dad's head dropped. His chest heaved in disappointment. The morning had indicated more hope. These numbers screamed intubate or watch her die. Her body couldn't get enough oxygen independently to keep her awake and alert. Her numbers were low even after being on oxygen. Dad wanted me to hear her voice, as he had heard once she woke from a full night's sleep with oxygen through a mask. He wanted me to be able to hear her say she loved me before we had to decide whether she wanted a tube down her throat that would take her ability to speak. He wanted her to be aware in order to make her own decision.

We asked a nurse to come speak to us, explain as much as she could, and requested the oxygen be given again to Mom so that perhaps we would have a chance to converse with her. The nurse was kind and patient but also loyal to the priorities in her profession. She gently suggested we let Mom rest after she put the oxygen back over her nose.

And so Dad and I trekked down those too clean, too bright hallways and returned to the waiting room with no good news and no clear plan. We did there what a waiting room is built for – we waited and we hoped, hoped that soon the most complicated decision Dad might ever have to make would somehow become simpler thanks to Mom's voice.

Waiting is a dangerous proposition when the patient's lungs are filling with a gas that is poison to the brain. At prolonged seventy percent oxygenation rates or worse, Mom stood risk of brain damage. She had probably reached those levels already en-route to the ER or waiting for the rural area ambulance to take her to Hays' ICU.

I cuddled Eli in the waiting room and smelled my baby instead of the too-clean hallways. I proudly displayed Eli's new skills of lifting his own head, rolling over, and sitting against my stomach to the family who came to be our support. Meanwhile, Mom couldn't walk, or sit, roll over, or even lift her own head due to the sedation and medical equipment.

My family went in, a few at a time, to pray over Mom, say the rosary, or to speak to her while she was not awake. A few visits later, in what must have been about two hours, my aunt Angie came back to tell us Mom was awake.

She lay in bed with her eyes open above dark rings. She smiled as we entered, an oxygen mask over her mouth and nose hooked to a BiPAP machine. She looked at me with a faint glimmer of joy, masked by the opaque haze of the drugs pumping into her system. I quickened my pace, all but running in the room to gently hug her shoulder. She patted me on the back with a hand attached to the monitors.

"I love you, Mom! I love you a lot." My words were emphatic, desperate, grateful, and blurted in one breath.

She smiled at me, said, "I love --" then she coughed. With effort, she brought her fist to her chest, then lifted the mask from her mouth. "I love you too."

Her words felt like a new beginning, a turning of a page, and, ominously, rang like the beginning of a final chapter. I nuzzled my nose into her chest, felt her skin against my face, and yearned for the warmth of her embrace when I was weak and she was strong. I wanted back the days when I would scrape my knee after falling from my bike and she would wipe away my tears and hold me in her capable arms. Her body was so different. She wasn't firm; she wasn't toned; she wasn't strong. Mom was bedridden and weak. I squinted my eyes closed tight, pushing away the tears. I fought the shudder that rose in my back, and I just held her, held on to what had given me life and so often had given me strength. I whimpered into her shoulder before I could catch myself.

"Eli's in the waiting room, Mom. He's not allowed to come in, but the family catching up with him." My voice cracked "He's grown so much."

Life seemed too fast. Why should I, at twenty-six, be leaving my infant in the waiting room to ask Mom any type of question about life support? In two weeks Mom was supposed to be living in my guest room, teaching me how to take care of my eight-week-old son. She was going to care for him as I returned to work. My best-laid plans were lying in a hospital bed in front of me. I wanted her to teach me how to do what she did so well. I drew in a deep breath, pursed my lips to stop the breath from escaping, then mumbled the only words that fit the moment: "I love you, Mom. I'll always love you."

It was then that I cried into my mother's arms.

She wrapped her arms around me, gripping one knuckle and pushing into my back. She whispered through her oxygen mask, "It'll be okay, honey. It'll be okay." I sobbed a little longer, prayed that God would let me have the strength my mother raised me to have, then felt Dad patting my back.

He held eye contact with Mom, kept his hand on my shoulder and said, "She's glad to see you awake, Mom. You seemed pretty out of it for a while."

Mom gave me a last pat on the back, and I stood straighter, watching the eye contact between my parents. She nodded at Dad's comment, her eyes seeming more glazed. She coughed again. Then she was gasping for air. The machines began to beep, and a nurse walked through the door. She refitted the oxygen mask, looked at the vital signs, and seemed unhappy. "Her CO_2 levels are still low. I don't think this mask is doing enough for her. She talked a while with the last visitors. She seems tired now."

Dad's eyes looked like a child's who spent six months of savings on a raffle for a pony and heard another boy's name announced. He was hurt, he was yearning, and he hadn't gotten his answer about intubation. He asked politely, almost meekly, "If we stay here quietly, can I hold her hand until she falls back asleep?"

The nurse looked at us both, back at the vitals, then said, "That sounds good for her; just try not to give her that type of stress again soon." She smiled, wrote something on her clipboard, put her hand on Dad's shoulder, then left. He sat next to Mom's bedside, telling her it would be okay, that with intubation she might gain enough strength to fight off the infection in her lungs, that she could get stronger soon. He told her to close her eyes and rest.

I sat in the recliner in the room, closing my eyes every few seconds, trying to let it sink in without sinking too deep. In about ten minutes, Mom was back to sleep. I left my father alone with her and headed to check on Eli.

When Dad returned to the waiting room about an hour later, he said Mom had woken up for a while, and they spoke about Eli. He said she wanted to try to get stronger so she could watch Eli grow up. Neither of them was ready to give up Jo Lyn's life so suddenly.

Daniel drove to Hays as soon as school finished. As a family, we discussed and gave permission for doctors to intubate Mom. Mom had clearly told Dad earlier in life that she wouldn't want to be resuscitated or live on a machine, but being intubated for a few days to fight an infection felt different. They'd never talked directly about intubation when discussing life support and final wishes. It was a murky area and hard to make a clear decision in the moment of being in a hospital in medical crisis. Mom wanted to live to see her grandson grow.

Intubation didn't last long. The lung infection wasn't improving, and intubation carried the risk of more infection. The doctor asked permission to perform a tracheotomy and insert the tubes directly through a surgical slit in her throat and hook Mom to a ventilator to combat the lung infection. He said that would improve her carbon dioxide levels. Since intubation, her weak and failed attempts to make it to the bathroom had stopped completely. Hooking her neck to a ventilator would mean she would be stuck to her equipment. What would her quality of life be if we allowed the life support? Would it be unto death? Would she fight the infection and be able to breathe again without life support? Was it worth it?

A tracheotomy would mean a long hospital recovery. We'd be stationary in Hays, Kansas, where no one in the family lived. We'd rather have transferred Mom to the hospital in Salina, where Dad could stay at our house and Daniel and I could resume a somewhat normal work schedule and get Eli to daycare before I had to go back to work. Transferring an ICU patient to another hospital is complicated, if not downright impossible. Without the tracheotomy, Mom was not stable enough to transport. After surgery, medication would have to stabilize her heart rate before she could leave the ICU. If it seemed she would be in the hospital for a week and then recover, living temporarily in a hotel in Hays would be okay.

Mom would be in the hospital at least as long as it took to fight her lung infection. Once her lungs were clear, she would need to recover enough strength to breathe on her own. In the meantime, the doctor sent off some of Mom's blood seeking to confirm she carried myotonic muscular dystrophy. He didn't have medical records on hand that diagnosed her with myotonic muscular dystrophy. The records of her initial diagnosis were in the National Archives since dad retired from the military. The doctor had never treated another patient with MMD, and he wanted to be sure she had the disease before he began to tackle treatment with an incurable disease.

Long-term care loomed as her best future option. Saying no to the tracheotomy meant the infection would overtake her lungs. Saying yes to the tracheotomy meant possibly having her live her final days hooked to a machine in a town where no one in the family lived. It felt like grasping at straws to hope Mom could come home after intubation to live her final days in a family home. Planning for a peaceful death felt preemptive. She had been healthy just last week: walking, talking, hosting a party for her ninety-year-old grandmother.

Dad cried, agonized, and prayed over the decision. We gave the doctors permission to perform the surgery.

Unfortunately, surgery is not as simple as just giving permission. The first day that the tracheotomy was scheduled, the surgeon was called to another small town around Hays to perform an emergency surgery, delaying the surgery a day. The next day, Mom's temperature rose due to increased infection. The doctors had to battle the infection and delay the surgery until later that night. Two nerve-racking and costly days after giving permission for life-support surgery, around six that night the surgery was complete.

The needle pricks on Mom's arms had blossomed into rose-hued patches of bruises. Her veins were hard to hit because her muscles were flaccid and moved with the needle. Her chapped lips had a half-inch sore because she was not drinking from a cup but an IV. She had bed sores from spending her whole day in bed unable to make it to the bathroom. When she was awake, if she were not sedated enough, she was in pain. If she were sedated enough, she didn't understand much, couldn't interact well, and slept often. In trying to save her life, her quality of life plummeted.

To alleviate the bedsores, she would be moved occasionally to the medical recliner in the room, which required at least two nurses for five minutes. Unfortunately, the recliner produced more discomfort than comfort. Those two nurses were busy and couldn't spend five minutes together easily. If Mom went to the chair, she had to sit there for a while. Some of the medicine caused adverse side effects, including vertigo. Sitting up would make her head spin and make her nauseous. She couldn't physically throw up, so she just sat there and felt bad.

In those two days, I wanted to say goodbye; I wanted to let it end quickly. I didn't want to have to continue living in a hotel with an infant away from my husband who still had to work. I didn't want visit a too-clean hospital too often and watch my mother suffer too much. Were the machines worth it? Were the blood blisters and chapped lips worth it?

It felt wrong. I felt wronged. I was angry at the irony of God giving me a new life just a month prior with Eli. Mom had been the first person in the room after Eli was born. Six weeks after that blessing of a new life, her quality of life declined so drastically that she might be better off dead than alive.

My emotions were complicated, but anger was limp and ineffectual. Being angry at God wasn't going to give me an answer. When I got to speak to Mom and hear words in response, I had wanted to be her strength and instead cried in her arms. I didn't want to fail Dad by reveling in anger at forces beyond my control. I was stressed, tightly wound, sleep-deprived, and emotional, but my family needed me. Dad needed me. He had always been a rock for me; I wanted to be that for him.

I'm not a rock. While I may have been able to hold my composure in the waiting room, most of the time with Mom, or during the car rides when I could nap, I didn't have much more than the rock veneer.

Mom's tracheotomy surgery was a success, but the doctors still had to combat her fever and tame the infection in her lungs. She rested on a cooling pad, had fans blowing on her, and was medicated with fever reducer. The incision on her neck was sore and tender. The gauze around her neck that was connected to the tubing chaffed her. She'd look at me with her lower lip gaping, her upper lip stretched back in fright or agony, and dry lips we could only dab with wet sponges. Her pupils would be wide and dark, the whites of her eyes magnified because her eyes were so opened, so searching, so panicked. When the fear hit, when her mind didn't know how to process the pain in her body or the machines attached to her, her eyes resembled a feral cat. Panic changed her features, and in her most instinctive moment of delirium, anxiety, and uncertainty, I wondered if her drugged mind could have even processed the feeling of regret in having the lifesaving surgery to put a tube in her throat.

Those days after the tracheotomy of combating the fever and infection were ugly. Seeking solace and a real night's sleep, the second day after her tracheotomy was the first time I went home. I might have tried to be a rock around my parents, tried to be strong for Dad and not cry in front of Mom, but when I got home to my husband, I just wanted to melt into a puddle in his arms and have him tell me it'd be okay. I cried to Daniel, told him I needed him, admitted how scared I was, how much it hurt to see the bruises on Mom's arms get bigger each day, and how hard it was to keep Eli in a waiting room or in a hotel or to constantly be near people that were trying to appear happy.

Being so scared and stressed, I wasn't aware of Daniel's needs and fears in a crisis he'd never been in before. He hadn't seen me much, since I was spending my maternity leave near the hospital, and he had returned to work at the beginning of the school year. He hadn't seen his son much either. I was wearing thin; he knew it, he was scared, and he needed his family too.

He said to me, "I need you too. Maybe you should stay here in Salina more often with Eli."

I railed my anger and fear against him. My job was to be by Mom every day in the hospital. How dare he want me somewhere besides with my dying mother? Why shouldn't Eli and I spend our time at the hospital? Eli needed to know my mother. I was blinded from my own needs, the stress and dangers of such a lifestyle with an infant son, and what was good for my family at that moment. All I could see was rage.

In looking out for his wife and son, Daniel unwittingly invited all my fear of the unknown to aim at him. I yelled curses at him. Fear overcame logic and my pores oozed with indignation.

Sometimes, the stress of having a loved one in the hospital is easier to deal with by being by his or her bedside than in your own home.

Eli's travel schedule was hectic. The hospital was hazardous to an infant. What Daniel said made sense. I should have listened to Daniel and calmly evaluated the needs of our family. Instead, I yelled angry insults. It wasn't easy to be married to me while Mom was in the hospital. I was trying to be so strong when I wasn't. Strength is a façade when a family member faces death, a veneer that comes off around the closest of friends or family. As strong as I wanted to seem next to Dad in Mom's hospital room, Daniel knew my weakness and helped carry me through it, even if I came at him kicking and screaming.

The next few days passed like the hectic Kansas wind. I returned to Hays the next day, sullen and angry at my husband for thinking I should be less consumed in the catastrophe around me. The quiet side of me, the part that didn't show up dressed for battle, was deeply grateful that he had pulled my head out of instinctual fight mode and showed he cared about me. Daniel was coming to the Hays hotel after work for the weekend. The way I was living wasn't a sustainable lifestyle for my eight-week-old son.

While Mom's temperature had subsided, she still had a lung infection. Grandma Jo had flown from New Mexico to visit her daughter, thinking this was goodbye. Jo Ann asked for us to have a hymnal for her. Mom was heavily sedated and scarcely awake. While she slept, either we had an iPod in a docking station playing Christian music or her mother would be by her bedside singing her favorite hymns like "In the Garden".

I walked into my mother's room to Grandma Jo singing "Amazing Grace." We hugged. She squeezed my hand, and kept singing. We stood there, hand in hand, singing "my chains are gone" as Mom lay sedated fighting for her life.

Later that day, Dad and I talked to the hospital social worker, who contacted insurance to advocate for a flight to take Mom to a long-term care facility as soon as she could leave the ICU. If Mom could survive without a ventilator, she could move to the hospital in my hometown; otherwise, she'd have to go to the largest city in the area to a facility that could provide long-term care with her on life-support.

Dad's brother, Rod Bartz, lived in Wichita and offered a friendly place to sleep, family to visit, and perhaps a return to some consistency. Dad told his other brother, Mike, that he should start looking for another skilled worker for Bartz Plumbing because he was going to take care of Mom long term.

If doctors could not combat the infection in her lungs, Mom would die in Hays. If she could regain enough strength to breathe without the ventilator, perhaps we could take her out of the hospital and give her care at home until her natural passing. Tricare approved a flight to a hospital in Wichita with long-term care facilities to move Mom out of the ICU, which was costing insurance about $30,000 a day.

Hospital flights are expensive, and once Mom was moved, insurance would not approve another flight to move her closer to family. If she went to Wichita, she would be there until her death or until she became strong enough to leave the hospital without ventilator support. Just a week ago her lungs were strong enough. It seemed her lungs could be again. What led to her steep decline? An aging body? Her genetic, incurable terminal disease? Pneumonia? Fourteen hour car trips? Could we get her back?

Mom needed out of the ICU. Her lips were cracking and bleeding, and she had an open wound on her backside. The overly clean smell and the hand sanitizer were there for a reason: an ICU contains potentially harmful germs, and long stays increase the risk of incurable germs like Staph infections. The health risks posed to healthy guests, who might carry those germs back to the waiting room and my infant son, were no small consideration. The decision to take Mom to Wichita was not what we had envisioned, but it was one of the only long-term care facilities able to support a patient on a ventilator. It seemed better than an ICU an hour from any family residence.

We gave the okay to move my mother to Wichita, knowing it might be the last place she ever went.

Chapter 13
When the Shadows of This Life

Mom's medicines had been adjusted to stabilize her heart rate for the flight, but the infection in her lungs persisted. Dad warned me that the medicinal cocktail Mom was receiving gave her vertigo and at times she woke disoriented and distressed. Her anxiety would get worse in a new environment because she wouldn't fully understand what was happening. He asked me to stay home for a few days so he could keep Mom calm and help her adjust to her new surroundings. Dad sensed how hectic the situation was for a new mother with a husband returning to work for the academic year. I spent some time trying to relax and enjoy the little moments of being a new parent with a crisis in my immediate proximity.

When I first went to the hospital in Wichita, I went with the man who had seen me cry the most and still offered his shoulder, my husband Daniel, and the person dependent on me to meet the needs his tears indicated, Eli. This hospital was larger, in the industrial part of town and tucked in between other businesses. Every piece of ground seemed paved and a slight coat of smog sat on the city. It may have been the carport entrance, or the color scheme – the lighting was less bright. This hospital wasn't like the newly built Hays ICU area with overly white walls and a too-clean smell; instead, the hallways seemed tight and dim. Everything felt older.

I clung to Daniel's hand in a not too white, not too clean elevator. I smiled at him nervously as we passed floor one, squeezed Eli against my chest past floor two, let out a sigh past floor three and let the silence nibble at my confidence four more floors. The waiting area was a constricted room with six chairs, two tables, and a window open to an expanse of flat roof.

Eli wasn't allowed in Mom's room. The 1,000 piece puzzles wouldn't keep Eli occupied. The nurses were nervous about Eli being on the seventh floor at all. Mom had pneumonia. How many other patients in long-term critical care had that or worse?

"Hey little girl." Dad greeted me with a term of simpler times.

"Hi. How's mom?" I asked anxiously.

"Good." He smiled reassuringly at me. "She's awake. Want to go see her?"

Daniel came over and rubbed my shoulder. He said "I can watch Eli so you and your dad can go together." That was the first time I felt comfortable since driving into the parking area. I tried to make the feeling last down the hallway.

The hospital room had floral print curtains with pink flowers on a green background dividing the room, though there was no other bed. The bottom half of the wall was painted the blue grey of a coming rainy day. Dull yellow cabinets accented the off-white upper walls, pragmatically adding storage space.

"Jo Lyn, your daughter is here to see you." Dad blared. I looked anywhere but at Mom, absorbing the room. Mom's eyes had been glossy for weeks. She tilted her head cockeyed in my direction. Her eyes focused above my head. Normally her eyes were a sky blue. Today they were the color was the grey of faded blue jeans washed a hundred times.

Dad spoke louder because her senses were dulled. Her hair had greyed visibly since she had entered the hospital; the solid streak of grey she had previously in her bangs had expanded so that now almost all the roots of her bangs were grey. Her mouth muscles pulled down in what now seemed a perpetual frown. Mom was older, tired.

She showed her happiness with her eyes. Her lips made more or less a square shape as she tried to smile. Her sheets were mostly on the bed, but the sheets weren't fitted and already had stains. The dark blue mattress showed through. I couldn't focus on my mother; in fact, with the age of everything and the dull color tone, it was like I heard the sound from the days when my phone had to dial into AOL to connect to the internet. I felt dismayed: The room didn't carry the energy of the living. Long term critical care embodied a frozen in time delay of waiting on death.

Constant noise brought my eyes to her ventilator machine. I followed the tubing to the fixture that dominated her throat, a large white tube connecting her, potentially for the rest of her life, to a machine. She had needles in her veins, a tan tube delivering food to her digestive system, and a monitor on her finger. Her machine beeped before my gaze returned to my half-smiling mother. The macabre looseness of her muscles limited my pleasure. I pushed my tongue to the top of my mouth and forced myself to swallow, trying to minimize the visible fright before I spoke.

"Hi, Mom," I said in a forcefully vivacious voice I learned from watching my father during crisis. "I'm glad to see you." I couldn't tell if I were lying.

She smiled in more of the orange slice shape we expect, then attempted to nod at me. Bruises lined the inside of her elbows from IVs lines. Her muscles didn't make it easy for the nurse to find her vein. Her body had been in one place all day. Her back lay lethargically submerged into the bed.

I had known Mom all my life. In that hospital room with so many tubes hooked to her, she felt like a stranger. I fingered the family pictures I'd brought. I tried to break the ice. Maybe showing Mom pictures of Eli at home would make us feel more ordinary. Sitting in the chair next to her bed, I smiled my best smile. I showed Mom a picture of Eli with his head raised off the floor. "Eli is growing strong. Look, Mom."

Mom's head tilted off center, and her glossy eyes tracked in the direction of the picture. "He can lift his head high." I pointed at his face and made an arc to the ground in the picture. "From here he rolls over by leaning his big head."

I watched her eyes as I told her about my best friend Michelle visiting Eli and how well they played together. Her eyes seemed fixated on some intangible floating object that occasionally moved about the room. I asked Dad for her glasses.

I put the frames on gently. Her plumper temples made it a tight fit. "Does that help any, Mom?"

She tried again to the look at the picture. She peered out at me under saggy brows, an apology in her billowy eyes. I smiled at her, held my hand over hers, and squeezed her fingers. I'd never felt so far from someone I could touch.

"It's okay, Mom. I'll tell you what it looks like. Eli is laying with his stomach on his Boppy, the pillow you bought me. He is in a onesie, a cute white one with little animals printed on it. His face is looking at me, his eyes wide." I glanced over at my mother, who was looking at the ceiling, smiling.

"He has his right elbow resting on the pillow. He's strong enough to prop himself up and hold his head up even without the pillow! Soon enough he might even be able to sit on his own." Her hospital gown hefted with her chest, and her head nodded more than once. She was laughing or coughing. I couldn't tell.

I continued talking through the pictures. A machine beeped; her oxygen was low. Her pale face turned toward the machine, but her eyes couldn't focus on that either. Her eyebrows raised in a look of bewilderment. Randy told her from the other side of the bed, "Your oxygen dropped a bit. You should be fine. That happens all the time."

Mom's face became more pained. She tried to go back to listening to me. She stared off more often. With effort, she raised the back of her hand to her forehead.

Dad came over and looked into her eyes. "Jo Lyn, are you dizzy?"

She raised her upper lip so that her two front teeth showed completely. She lifted her nose slightly as a 'yes.' He took off her glasses and told her to close her eyes.

"Vertigo," he said tremulously. "Her medicine makes her head spin, and then her best answer is sleep." I quietly slumped back into the chair by her bed with my hand around her thumb. Her hand was taken by an IV and covered in bruises. The story went unfinished.

She couldn't talk, couldn't breathe on her own, had blunted senses, and experienced vertigo regularly as a side effect of the medicine. I wanted my mother, needed her, and didn't want to lose her while learning to be a mother myself. It was painful to show her pictures she couldn't see, but that pain felt good because it meant she wasn't dead, or wasn't completely dead, or there was hope, or -- well, at least I had gotten to talk to her.

I trudged to the waiting room after Mom fell asleep. Silently, I walked in and grabbed my son. I held Eli against my chest, sobbing into his soft cheeks. Daniel placed his hand on my back, unsure of what to say, I held my face close to Eli's because next to him was where I felt closest to what was supposed to happen in the natural course of life.

I wept and murmured a frantic whisper: "God, don't let her live here long. Thy will be done, but take her peacefully or heal her quickly."

"This is painful" I snorted out. To Daniel I cried the tears I suppressed around anyone else. I sobbed until Daniel went to tell Dad we were going so Eli and I could rest. I felt distant, as if my ambition for getting Mom home had glazed over and my pain was inaccessible. I floated in a false calm that comes after deep sorrow.

I didn't cry on the way home.

I would be in Wichita for twelve of the next fourteen days. Sometimes I would drive down alone and return that night, sometimes I would catch a ride and bring Eli, sometimes I would go stay the weekend and sleep in my uncle Rod's house in Wichita, and sometimes my husband would go with me. Perhaps the intense love felt in the midst of intense sorrow was addictive.

About ten days after Mom's transfer flight, I traveled to Wichita with my two aunts who live near me in Salina. Bedsores made Mom uncomfortable in the only location she was strong enough to be, her bed. The infection in her lungs had receded, the fact that she had an open wound on her back was complicated by not being able to walk to the bathroom. Her muscles had weakened even further, and if we were ever to get her out of the hospital, strength therapy was necessary. A therapy chair would relieve the bed sores and to allow Mom to exercise. Mom's first excursion in the therapy chair lasted less than thirty minutes. Sitting up induced vertigo, and her spinning head made sitting intolerable. Progress was slow.

Aunt Karla offered to take the first shift entertaining Eli in the waiting room. I ventured to Mom's room alone. The same worn-out curtains were my first greeting, followed by the view of the tarred roof from the window. Dad stood in a tourist shirt from Alcatraz Prison, ironically dressed in prisoner stripes. I didn't notice Mom in the chair until I peeked around the corner near the curtains. She sat reclining in a worn large blue chair with her sizable ruffled hospital gown sagging on her shoulders.

She was still connected to at least three different machines: her ventilator, the feeding tube, and her IVs. How comfortable could she be? The therapy chair had torn corners and an ill-fitting sheet. At any second, her body might spoil the moment. If she had to go to the bathroom, she'd have to go in the chair then wait for someone to move and clean her. Nothing was easy once her life depended on a machine.

Trying to hide my thoughts, I grinned at Mom. "Hi, Mom. How are you today?" I had carried in a white board and marker to see if she could write. I noticed she wasn't wearing her glasses. I tucked the white board away under my arm.

He lips stretched across her cheeks, and she lifted her hand and turned her wrist, indicating 'so-so'. Dad, however, was excited. "Jo Lyn, tell Darcy what you just gave Angie." I looked dubiously toward her. Mom couldn't tell me much at this point. She looked at me with a tilted head, smiled, and shifted like she was laughing. Then she put both arms out in front of her as if embracing the air and mouthed two words: 'a hug.' My heart flittered. Could she hug me? Was there hope she would regain abilities she had lost? Could this ragged therapy chair give me back my mother?

I sat the white board on her bed. Angie had pulled out the camera I handed her in the waiting room. Dad showed me a video on his phone of how Mom had given him an encircling embrace, how she even squeezed his back with her arms wrapped around him. She gave him hope.

Brisk goosebumps rose below my short sleeves as I strode toward Mom. A real 'wrap her arms around me' embrace would restore a part of the mom I had lost, maybe give me the hope Dad seemed to have. I stood in front of her chair, leaned in and put my arms under Mom's. Her left hand went under my shoulder, pushing up against my armpit. Her right arm clasped around my arm just beneath my shoulder.

Dad coached from his chair. "Wrap your arms around her. There you go." He sounded like the man who coached my softball team when I was five. "C'mon, let me have the other hand. You got the other hand up there too?"

Angie, watching from behind the camera, said, "Yep." I felt a silly, blissful pride. My mother's hands were on my shoulder and in my arm pit. That was more physical affection from her than I'd gotten in a month. I was a child in the embrace of my mother. I yearned for the days I'd sit in her lap and rest my head on her soft neck, when I could feel the warmth of her body surround my chest, when she could run and play with me, when she would carry me off to my bed – when she could breathe.

The ventilator tube rubbed my chin as Mom squeezed my arm. I tried to dig my head into her chest. "There you go." Dad whispered over my shoulder. This was my mother, here was my hope, and I wanted more: I wanted to feel her full embrace; I wanted her to be able to carry Eli to his bed; I wanted to take her home. My breath became deeper. I turned to face her. I kissed her on the cheek. I looked her in the eyes, inches from her face, and I said, "I love you." She rubbed my arm, patting me on the back. She pursed her lips, and I kissed my mother. It was then I rested my head on her shoulder and bawled.

I had my mother; we had made progress. Dad cheered her on. Yet the hope was in a dispirited old chair, and the hug was hampered by an obtrusive ventilator tube. She had patted my back; she had not embraced. I had more than I had a week ago, but I did not have enough of my mother to help me raise Eli. I cried in Mom's arms, cried the type of tears a daughter can only give to her dying mother.

That moment was a drop of rain in a desert that was once fruitful ground. Dad requested Mom receive a mitigated dose of her pain medication so she could be more aware. Next time I arrived, she was more aware and responsive than she had been the past few days.

Mom's hand coordination had improved; she had patted my back. I wanted to see if she could write on the whiteboard. I handed the pen to her and asked if she could write her name. Her hand awkwardly grasped the marker, trembling and unsteady. She brought the pen to the board and drew something of a horizontal straight line. Then she attempted to lift her pen to begin the downward stroke of the J and covered half the board in a series of zig-zagged lines. She huffed and looked at me dejectedly. She wasn't able.

She couldn't read what I wrote on the board either. So again, I talked to her rather than with her, telling her stories of what Eli was doing, talking about the pictures I had brought, and reliving old memories. While I was there, we uploaded the videos of her to Facebook, asked for visitors to come, called for prayers, and ordered an extra-large keyboard to use with a text-reading voice. I was desperate to communicate with her. I left with hope and a hug but no sure answers, and only a memory of her voice.

Back in Salina, Daniel had returned to teaching and coaching soccer. He was working from about 6:30 a.m. to 6:30 p.m. I saw him rarely; when I did, I saw him through blood-shot eyes and often wanted to discourse about the tragedy around me. Daniel, too, was worn out during the adjustment from the pace of a teacher's summer to a coach's sixty-hour work week. I was exhausted from going to the hospital constantly and crying every day. I would go to the hospital seeking in my heart something that couldn't fully be mine anymore. I came home unfulfilled. Now that the infection was gone, I was still hopeful that the hospital staff might get her to sit in a therapy chair to ease her bed sores, or that she may become strong enough to breathe without a ventilator, or that she may relearn sign language or be able to type on an oversized keyboard, but the odds were long. Each trip began with the hope Mom might relearn and ended with the feeling I'd lost so much of my mother.

My heart ached. My motherly instincts dominated any feelings left over after the hurt. Eli was my refuge, a growing boy who needed me. I devoted myself to Eli. I cuddled him, stroked his face, dawdled on every development or breakthrough, and buoyed myself in the juxtaposition of his potential compared to Mom's drastic degeneration. I was an attentive mother while Mom was in the hospital. I was not an attentive wife.

I was exhausted, depressed, addicted to the pain of seeing Mom. One night I dreamed that I was being chased and running along the rooftop of the hospital outside Mom's window. It was dark, and whoever was chasing me wanted to bring about death. If I could get to Mom before my assailant caught me, I'd be safe. I ran and leaped over a barrier on the roof and spilled the carpet bag I was carrying, exposing my 'baggage': the arms and legs of my deceased brother, Dustin. In the dream I scrambled to pick up the limbs, knowing it meant I had lost ground in escaping. I sat on the roof and cried as I recollected each appendage and placed it back in the bag. My assailant jumped into view from another part of the roof, and I ran away with the bag unzipped. I was about to reach the window of Mom's hospital room when my assailant put his hand on my shoulder, and I woke up with tears streaming down my face. The stress had sunk into my spirit, and even my dreams were edgy. I was in chaos; Daniel was married to an overstressed mess.

One weekday after I came home from visiting the Wichita hospital, I was emotionally drained, numb, and listless. I had taken Eli with me, so I quietly laid him in his crib. As I watched him sleep, I sighed heavily then curled up near the foot of his bed, rested my head on my arms near his legs, and let my chest pulse with silent tears. It was already ten-thirty. I was set to return to work that next week teaching full-time.

Daniel was grading papers on the couch when I trudged out of Eli's room. I barely noticed. I walked to the bathroom, silently cried some more, tried to wash the tears off my face, then went into the living room to kiss Daniel good night.

He didn't have a paper to grade in his hand when I leaned in. I absently kissed his forehead, without passion, without presence. He looked at me from the corner of his eyes, his hands crossed on his lap. His lips pursed together; his brows burrowed slightly. He had something to say. The cavernous emptiness inside me made it feel like all the weight of my body was inside the bones at the bottom of my back. I didn't want to talk.

I heard my voice reverberate inside my ears, "I'm exhausted. I'm going to bed." He tried to stare into my eyes. I avoided his gaze, turning my head to look down the hallway towards the bedroom. He put his hand around my own. I squeezed his hand once, more in an attempt to end the gesture than to return it. I smiled at him weakly, barely lifting the edges of my lips, not letting the smile touch my eyes. I said, "I love you" trying to end the conversation.

I started to walk towards the bedroom. I put my hand out to reach for the door knob.

"Darcy, I'm lonely."

The exhaustion sitting in my lower back elevated to a fear that shook my spine. I sighed, knowing how desperately I wanted to sleep the rest of that day away. In a bone-weary voice, I said, "I can't talk, Daniel. I'm just so tired."

"You've been gone every evening this week. Half the time you take my son with you. I saw you both every day over the summer, and now, unless we are both crying in some hospital that traps our son in that small waiting room, I don't get to see you. I need you. You're my best friend."

His voice held on to the edge of panic. He was afraid -- afraid of the situation, afraid of losing his mother-in-law, afraid of losing his wife to grief, unsure of how to transition from summer break to being a new father working more than sixty hours a week. He was afraid of being alone while chaos swirled around our family life. I sensed it in his distressed voice, but I didn't have the energy to be his friend right then.

Without even glancing in his direction, I curtly responded in self-preservation, "Daniel, don't be selfish during the hardest time of my life. I need sleep. I can't talk tonight. Karla is picking me and Eli up at seven in the morning to go visit my mom." My voice was both faint-hearted and perturbed. "Just let me go to bed."

He had left the couch and must have walked silently, or I must have been so self-absorbed, but I didn't notice him at first when he stepped forward and put a hand on my hip. His voice was grim, the type of flatness that comes when fears aren't relieved but instead greeted by insult. "Darcy, it isn't selfish. You haven't been here at all, and when you have, you're just surviving. I don't want to lose your mother and, by consequence, my wife. This isn't the way we want to live; this isn't why we became parents. You have to spend more time with me than you have been." His tone was adamant but caring. "We can't go on this way. I feel alone."

Perturbed, I pushed away his hand and glared at him in indignation. I raised my voice and spoke in an imperious tone. "My mother is dying, Daniel!" I yelled at him. "I swear you're the most selfish person I've ever met. You drag me down in trying to make yourself happy!" Averting my eyes and staring at the floor, I almost pleaded. "I need my sleep. I'm sorry we haven't talked in a while. Please, just leave me alone."

I ignored his reflection in our mirror. I walked quickly to my side of the bed and went under the covers without changing for bed. Daniel stood in the doorway. "Darcy, I've cooked my own dinners, eaten alone, done the dishes, then watched TV until you come home exhausted and upset the last four days. What am I supposed to do? Just accept that your mother's situation means I lose my family? I can't do that."

He was trying to divert the only precious time I had left with Mom. My cheeks were hot, and my words spewed from lips under a nose runny from crying so often. I sat up in bed and threw off the cover. "Damnit, you just don't get it. This isn't about you! Why don't you take more time off and come with me? Why can't you just get that I need to be there?"

His eyes held sympathy, which didn't calm my hostile heart. "Are you really obligated to be there so often, Darcy? She's been in the hospital almost two months. You've spent so many days there, driving on the road. The costs are starting to pile up, not just the money. Look at how quick you snapped at me. This isn't good for our marriage. It can't be good for Eli. We all have to make sacrifices." He paused, but carefully queried, "Are you making the right ones?"

I sobbed, indignant and resigned. "She's dying, Daniel. I've already lost my brother. I can't lose my mom." I buried my eyes in my hands, yearning for a slumber that would quiet my restless mind. "What do you want me to do?"

He sat on the bed next to me, embracing my shoulder and putting his hand on mine. "Darcy, you can't decide whether or not you lose your mother. You can't save her by being at her bedside. She can never take care of Eli. It isn't going to happen. But don't cut your heart off from me in the middle of all this." His lightened tone carried optimism. "Who knows, it could be another year before she passes."

He leaned in gently, staring kindly into seething eyes. "We need each other, Darcy, even when it hurts." He tenderly kissed my lips. "We have to figure something out. What you're doing isn't sustainable."

I sighed, and finally the panic that had risen from the feebleness in my back to the constriction in my chest heaved into a release of the tension to someone who understood. I wrapped my arms around his neck and buried my face into his chest, wetting his shirt with my tears and muttered breathlessly, "It won't be a year..."

He held me until I fell asleep, listening to my fears, and when his alarm went off that morning to get ready for work, we were cuddled under the covers in our day-old clothes. He lightly kissed me as a goodbye and let me drift back to sleep. I returned it passionately. He had saved my sanity when I bordered on sullen servitude to the sorrow.

I called Karla and let her know I'd only be going to Wichita if we could be back before Daniel would get off of work. I told Dad that next week, when I returned to work, I wouldn't come during the weekdays, that I had to spend time with my husband and son in our home. Next Friday I'd see him with Daniel and Eli. My heart broke when I told him that I wouldn't be suffering every day by Mom's side as he would be, but it gave my sensibilities the chance to start mending.

I went back to work, trying to put my passion into my students. I missed visiting my parents daily, but I cooked meals, cleaned house, spent time with Eli where we weren't potentially near pneumonia or other dangerous infections in a critical care wing, and ate dinner with my husband at the dinner table. I went to visit my parents with Daniel on the weekend, staying overnight with my uncle Rod in Wichita. It felt much better to be there with my husband – life was more manageable; balance was in reach.

We had an outpouring of visitors on the weekend. Mom wasn't always able to greet the visitors with a smile, and sometimes our friends simply conversed with Dad and me in the waiting room as she slept, but those visits meant so much. It helped avoid isolation during a fight in which our most necessary allies were heartless machines and the twenty-four hour cycle of a busy hospital staff. In my absence, I'd post pictures to Facebook and ask our family friends to visit my parents and help us through the situation. Those visits meant the most to Dad when I wasn't there. I'd send pictures in the mail each day with a note written in extra-large letters on the back, which gave him ten to fifteen minutes of new conversation every day. But he began to find that Mom would forget what was on the pictures from day to day. Every day he showed her every picture in the stack and read every word on the back.

In one picture session, Mom knew me, Daniel, and Eli but couldn't name Dustin when I showed her an older picture. Her oxygen levels had dipped below 70% oxidation enough that the effects were palpable.

Mom had lost the ability to count, to write, to read, to see well, to fully follow in-depth conversations, didn't remember her sign language alphabet, and at times didn't remember her son's image. Whether by the natural course of her medical condition or the heavy sedatives she was on, Mom was not capable of many things she once had been.

Once, after being in the hospital for over a month and a half, when everyone else had left the room for lunch and I wanted to stay with Mom, she mouthed to me 'What's wrong with me?' When she would ask Dad this question in front of me, he would answer, "Nothing, dear, you are just the way God made you, and I love you through and through." She would half smile, roll her eyes at him, and go on. She asked me alone because she wanted an answer.

She'd been told by Dad, by doctors, but never by me. She knew. Part of her knew, or at least, mom as she was two months ago would have known. But she didn't know in that moment. She wanted me to tell her. I knew why Dad told her nothing was wrong. I considered lying.

I grasped her hand with both of my own, looked into her eyes and asked, "You don't know why you are in the hospital this morning?" She looked at my hands in a gesture something like shame, shook her head, then mouthed 'Why?' I inhaled deeply. Then I told her everything I knew.

"You remember the boy in the picture, your son Dustin? You have the same disease he did, myotonic muscular dystrophy." She peered through eyes that would have been wide if she weren't trying to squint with weak muscles in an attempt to understand. I walked over to the windowsill and grabbed the picture of Dustin. I pointed to his wheelchair. "Dustin's muscles were weaker because of his disease, so he used his wheelchair. During puberty, his heart couldn't support his body's growth." I held her hand again and massaged the back of her hand with my thumb. "You remember Dustin, don't you?"

She nodded yes and looked left then right, processing what I had said. Then she mouthed "what about me," wanting to know why she was there. "Well, Mom, we thought you were sick in New Mexico because of the mountains or allergies, but what was really happening was that your brain wasn't getting enough oxygen. Your oxygen levels have been helped by the ventilator, but without it, your body would fail and you'd run out of oxygen. Your heart's still good, Mom, but your body isn't strong enough to give you a full breath of air on its own."

Her eyes were locked on mine, afraid but not surprised -- aware but not fully understanding. She asked me, 'Will it get better?' I pushed my lips together, opened my mouth, closed it, pushed air out my nose, and thought. I closed my eyes for composure, opened them, and gave a compassionate, brittle smile. I wanted to tell her everything I knew. I wanted her to be able to understand. I wanted her to be in control of where her life went from here. I wanted to be able to talk to my mother. Her ability to ask a related series of questions suggested she could understand. She deserved to hear what I knew, even if she wouldn't fully understand, even if it would hurt.

"Mom, they've been fighting an infection in your lungs since Dad first took you to the hospital in Larned. The hospital staff beat the infection, but by that time your body had been in a bed and not moving much for a month. The myotonic dystrophy won't stop weakening your muscles. Your disease has no cure. They gave Dustin steroids to help his body grow stronger, but he was younger, and I don't think your heart could handle steroids. If you can regain enough strength to breathe on your own again, they can start weaning you off the ventilator, but it wears you out pretty bad when they lower your oxygen. They haven't tried removing the ventilator in about a week."

Her expression wilted, either in surprise or distress or as a sign that her awareness and control were lessening. She took her open hand to her chest and tried to breathe in deep. She wanted to feel how much her chest moved. It wasn't much.

Then my mother asked me the hardest question, mouthing 'Do I die here?'

I squeezed her hand and sighed heavily. "Dad has been trying really hard to get you to our house... but Mom, they can't let you leave the hospital with a ventilator. We'd have to get you transitioned to nose oxygen for that to happen." I paused and admired her face. I recalled her muscles firm. She once had high cheekbones and sun-kissed skin. The fluids injected into her bloated her features. She looked something between the mother of my memories and a dead body ashore after a tsunami. Modern medicine had distorted the face I knew.

"There is a good chance you spend your last days here, Mother. They might be able to make your last days last a little longer." I looked away in shame, turning my head right at the rip in the worn-out therapy chair. I needed to know. "Do you like it here? Do you want to be on the machines?"

She too moved her head over to look at the chair, right next to her heart rate monitor. She mouthed 'home,' letting her top lip rest heavily on the bottom. I blinked at the tears welling in my eyes.

"We'll try, Mom; we'll try. You and Dad can live with me and Daniel, and we can take shifts taking care of you." I hugged her, careful not to get in the way of any wires attached to her, and nuzzled my cheek into her soft arms.

When we let go, she weakly joined her hands by crossing her two thumbs and flapping her hands like a butterfly. I smiled. Dustin had liked butterflies. They were a symbol of hope. She was saying more than that. "You're making a butterfly, Mom."

She smiled and nodded yes. Then she mouthed something I didn't understand. "Go away? You want me to give you a break?"

Mom pushed her lips together and turned her head in frustration and mouthed 'no' with enough emotional emphasis to be clear. She mouthed, again, 'fly away.' I understood. She was referencing the hymn "I'll Fly Away," which begins with the line "Some bright morning when this life is over, I'll fly away. To that home on God's celestial shore, I'll fly away." Mom was telling me that the home she wanted to go to was in heaven. My mother had told me she was ready to die.

"You're ready to fly away, huh, Mom?" She nodded, smiled, then put her hand on my arm and patted, comforting me when it was her who was approaching the end of life.

***

Dad had wanted to give Mom's family from New Mexico the chance to visit. He had felt for a while that Mom would not regain enough strength to leave the room she was tied to by three different machines. Her nights were restless, and she woke up disoriented, in pain, or forgetting where she was. Once in her hysteria, she forgot him. The staff asked him to leave that night, and for once in that month, he slept in a real bed at his brother's house.

He kept cheering, kept hoping, but he saw the signs. He was there every day: he knew she wasn't gaining sustainable vitality, even if there were little gains. He did want to bide the time though, to see if Jo Lyn seeing her mother again would give her enough fight, if something miraculous would happen in the next week or so that might give Mom the chance to expire in the home of her family. Dad wanted to get her to a bed he could climb into and lie next to her on as she drew her last breaths, maybe even a place where he could take care of her for a few years, a few months: anything would have been better than dying in the care of strangers.

At first, I wondered whether such a decision -- to discontinue life support -- was legal to make with someone who could not speak and who had not signed a 'Do Not Resuscitate' card before losing her ability to write or be understood. We had tried to reteach her how to sign her name to give power of attorney to my father to get her flown to Wichita, which she ended up signing with a shaky X. The decisions weren't simple nor mine to make.

Dad took some time to ponder the time limits of life. He wanted to speak to Mom about her choice on another day when she was coherent enough to ask multiple questions and understand the responses. His body posture slumped. The sluggish look in his eyes indicated he was terrified. What I told Dad about Mom wanting to "Fly Away Home" disappointed the part of him that was still cheering for recovery. He still didn't want to believe a genetic disease could take his son in thirteen years and his wife in fifty-one.

All Dad's sisters were in town. Angela played 'thumb wars' with Mom, using the same voice she used with children as a daycare provider, and my mother enjoyed it, even acted like a rascal by sticking her tongue out. Theresa painted Mom's fingernails, treating Mom like a lady when Jo Lyn had been able to wear nothing but a hospital gown for over a month. My grandma Carol massaged Mom's hands, rubbed her arms, and told her what a terrific job she had done as a mother and wife. Aunt Karla brought hair pins and makeup. They treated Mom like a successful matriarch, a woman who deserved love and pampering after a job well done.

I cried when I told Angie how thankful I was for the sisters coming and giving my mother such positive attention. She insisted, "I know she's your mother, and that makes you want to thank me, but she's my sister too. I love her."

She didn't say sister-in-law. She wasn't there for her brother. She genuinely loved my mother. They all did, and they showed it through simple acts of kindness and purposeful caring.

Those moments exemplify one of the most beautiful aspects of the human condition – women's ability to build each other's confidence and self-worth, even when the recipient sits on her deathbed in a hospital gown.

I updated friends and family of Mom's decision on Facebook with a call for visitors to ease her transition to her final days. Part of it read:

I cannot express how much gratitude I have towards those who have visited my mother, sent cards, or prayed for my family. Every expression of love and good will is so much more meaningful when we know that we, or someone we care deeply about, will soon no longer walk the Earth. God has plans in what has been happening, and my mother has experienced an abundance of love and support and been able to smile, hug, and appreciate many wonderful people in her life.

What my mother faces is beyond my capacity for imagining. Part of me wants to drop everything and hold her hand every second from now until she passes quietly into the good night. I have a 10 week old son and a teaching job and can't quite do that. My father has been at my mother's side constantly. Tonight he is taking a break from the hospital to hug Eli and me and sleep at our house. My mother, while ready, will certainly experience some fear, some loneliness. She can't talk on the phone. She can't write letters. Visitors mean so much to her. If you care for my mother and want closure, please come visit her. Send a card and my father will read it to her. Send a Facebook message and we will share it. Come hold her hand and let her know her life was good, worthwhile, and impactful. My mother is ready to go to God and waiting to say good bye to her mother, brother, and sister. If you can make that waiting easier in anyway, I thank you from the bottom of my heart.

Many friends responded to that post and came to visit, making the time until Mom's family arrived easier to bear. Mom's family wanted to come be together one last time with her, but it would take a few days to organize, meet, and drive to Kansas. My cousin Tanya and her husband Jay were the first to arrive. My uncle Donald Woodard drove to pick up his sister, Donna Tash, gathered my grandmother Jo Ann Talley in New Mexico, and covered five states to reach his sister. Mom's family made great sacrifices, taking off work and incurring travel expenses, to visit the hospital and spend time with mom.

Mom was so elated to finally see her family. I may not be able to fathom what it's like to lay on in a hospital bed wanting release from a machine that provides a quality of life lower than anything you were once accustomed to, but because of Mom's face and the visible uplift of her chest, I can imagine the extreme joy that comes when you are waiting on death and you get the chance to see, for the last time, some of the most important people in your life.

Dad was hoping the joy from seeing family would give her strength to recover. Mom was indeed elated, but elation came with a price. She was so overjoyed when she saw her brother that she cried instantly, visible tears that must have hurt her body because she convulsed and had tightly-closed eyes. She wanted to be around her family, wanted to talk with them. She smiled more, moved more, and didn't want to sleep while they were in the room. Mom was exhausted a few hours after her family arrived.

The ventilator tube had rubbed sore spots on her neck, and swiveling her head to look at more than one person in the room at a time caused pain. The pain caused shame, and the tiredness embarrassed her. She felt so guilty when she would go to the bathroom in her bed and the nurses would clear everyone out. Mom wanted to be around her family, and while she enjoyed their presence, she didn't want to be around them like this: unable to speak, unable to control her own body, unable to breathe on her own, unable to hold her focus or remember everything they talked about happening in the past. She didn't want her family to be visiting a hospital from over a thousand miles away and have her memory fail her. She cherished the moments she was strong enough to enjoy, but she didn't want to be that way.

As Mom tired near the end of the first visit, Grandma Jo wanted to sing hymns. We gave them time alone so a mother could sing her daughter to sleep one of the last times in her life. Mom closed her eyes and relaxed, trusting my grandmother to sing hymns of praise and bathing in the comfort of the voice she had known since being in the womb. Mom slept, or tried to the entire rest of the day. After everyone but Dad had gone home, Mom had a restless, painful night and wasn't easy to manage by the hospital staff.

The next day when she was awake, alert and calm, the family gathered to talk about pictures and memories. Grandma Jo was standing next to Mom's bed, dressed in a western blouse reminiscent of her New Mexico roots with red and gray stripes, speckled like the desert sand. Her hair was short and curly, grayed with age beyond her dying daughter's years. Her face was kind but more stressed than tender. She took off work and spent savings to visit her dying daughter in the hospital for a second time. Grandma Jo held the pictures I had written on and sent in the mail each day. Mom held a photo in her hand, but she didn't look at it. Instead, she tried to speak to her mother. Grandma Jo leaned in, trying to understand. She put her ear next to Mom's mouth. "Huh?" She said with a bit of a southern twang.

Mom repeated something in her ear. Grandma Jo raised her head and asked, "Flag?" Mom moved her hand in a wave motion.

The nurse aide who had worked with Mom four days a week for her entire stay piped in "Flag waves!" as if she had solved the mystery. Mom repeated the wave motion, but at the end of it, lifted her palm high and flat, ending the wave in some type of exit.

Grandma gave another attempt, still not understanding. "Waves like a flag?" she asked her daughter. I knew what Mom was trying to tell her mother, but it was her place to do the telling. It needed to come from her.

Then, mom clearly mouthed the word 'home.' I said two words, simply, and in the form of a question, "Fly away?"

My grandmother's back rose, and she no longer leaned in towards Mom's mouth. "Ohh," she exclaimed. "Fly away home. Okay." Mom dropped her hand quickly, relieved to be done with the effort. Jo Ann looked her other daughter, Donna, in the eyes and repeated the motion of a hand waving as if riding the waves. "Fly away home."

Donna understood at the same time. "Fly away home – that's what that meant."

Mom looked at me while her mother looked away, a split second of recognition in a glance that said she had accomplished what she had wanted. She was glad I understood. She seeped deeper into her pillow.

Grandma pointed at her healthy daughter. "Okay, that's fly away home."

Dad asked, "Were you telling the nurse last night to fly away home?'

Grandma had seen the hand signal before. She replied, "No, we were talking about a song," referring to her hymn singing experience from the day before.

Donna has been a nurse for many years. "She says that when the nurse was poking her last night, what she wanted to say was that she 'just wanted to fly away home.' Right, Jody?"

Mom looked at Donna and nodded her head in agreement.

Grandma argued in the tone of a mother. "Noooo."

Donna repeated her idea, knowing what it was like to be a nurse poking a patient. "Yes, that's what she was saying." Donna's voice pitched up with the excitement of figuring out a puzzle. "When he was poking her, instead of being mean to him, she told him she just wanted to fly away."

Grandmother said, "Well, that's what she was telling me yesterday when we were trying to find songs."

My heart heaved. Mom had been giving her message of readiness to meet her maker to me, her mother, her sister, and the nurse. She wanted us to listen; she was ready to be heard. She looked intently at her mother, her eyes moving slowly as the conversation went back and forth between her sister and her mother. I wondered how much of what her family said she understood. I hoped her family could come to understand. She had told them she was ready to die.

Chapter 14
Waiting

We had told the doctors of Mom's decision, had her sign her name with an X on paperwork she could only slightly comprehend, and hoped we could 'pull the plug' while her family was still in town. Mom would have to wait at least a week before they could honor her request to 'fly away' to her Savior and a pain-free existence. My aunt and uncle had to return to their work and their families, and my grandmother, though she wanted to stay, would have to ride back with them and back to her obligations. Mom would have to endure her last few days without her family because her choice and free will became complicated legal matters once she was connected to a life-sustaining machine and lost the ability to speak.

September 20 the doctor would have the time to remove the tracheotomy from Mom's neck. Hopefully she could spend her last hours in a comfortable room in hospice care. Maybe we would be able to speak with her again without the tube in her neck. Dad wanted to crawl into Mom's bed and let her drift to her rest holding his hand while he lay next to her. The nurse smiled when we said such things and politely nodded her head.

Every minute with Mom was ticking away to a known end. Her disease had no cure, her medicine had debilitating side effects, and her body hurt. Life passed in minutes. Her brain was befuddled, her memory drifting, as more and more often her oxygenation went past the point of possible brain damage. Wanting to spend every possible minute with Mom, I took that last week off of work and stayed in Wichita with Dad. During the last two nights of her life on earth I slept on a mat in her hospital room.

My mat was in the corner, a large blue fold-up with the same type of tears as the therapy chair. I slept in sweats and a long sleeve t-shirt and was still cold. Dad gave me his pillow. He said he would sleep in the hospital, but he didn't. He sat in the chair next to her bed, held her hand, prayed, sang her songs, and tried to comfort her each time she woke delirious. The life partner he had lived with over thirty years had less than 48 hours left.

He had been giving his life to her, constantly at her side during her time in the hospital, and now he sat on a precipice, knowing he was losing the love of his life. Part of his life was fading; another member of his family was going to be dancing in heaven but no longer with him. That night was ominous, intense, and poignant.

My heart was anxious as I lay on the type of mat I had slept on in kindergarten, when Mom could still ride bikes with me and read me into sleep. I marveled at the chaos that was her life each time an alarm beeped to indicate her oxygen levels were critical, or that her monitor was no longer on her finger, or that her body was tensing because it need to pass gas. Between beeps I would drift off to sleep, only to be awakened by footsteps coming for routine hourly checks, talk between staff on shift changes, or Dad talking to Mom to ease her back to sleep.

In the deepest part of her mind, Mom knew she was ready to fly away home and join her son in heaven, leaving behind the pain of the earthly body and the trap of machines that prolonged her death. But each time she woke up, she was scared. Perhaps she expected to be in her own bed, didn't know why there was a tube in her neck, or knew there was a needle to come. Like a cat dangling over the water, she lived always fearing the plunge, never sure of her footing, and constantly tense. Mom wanted to be as aware as possible during her final hours, so we had asked the staff to avoid sedating her. Otherwise, she would have been incapable of conversation. Perhaps she would forget what she had told her mother or what had happened to put her in this state. The lack of sedation meant she was restless until about three in the morning. Dad tried to guide her in each step and reassure her.

I cried silently on the mat. I trusted God to take care of her eternal fate, but I feared for Dad once he lost this bastion of purpose in taking care of his wife. I feared for myself, raising a child of my own without a mother to ask advice from. The thing I feared least was my mother's body ceasing to draw breath. I feared the uncertainties of my life after her death. For her, death was a release.

When I woke in the morning to the sun drifting in through the window, another shift nurse entered the room. My shoulders were sore, like the floor had melded with the mat and my spine. Squinting out the window toward the sun let fear squeeze around my heart again; Mom's clock was setting as the sun was rising. I went to the bathroom to wash the dried tears from my face and confronted a mirror image of a bedraggled woman, ten years older than she was – someone staring death in the face. I washed, held my hand over my mouth, and let out a sigh – a sigh of preparation for a desired, yet dreaded, outcome.

In about twenty-four hours, Mom's life support would be removed, and her muscles, degenerated by MMD, would be given one chance to sustain her. My eyes were the blue of a still-clear pond, my eye sockets hollow and deep, cheeks puffy, and there was a line down my face from sleeping on a plastic mat. I didn't smile at my reflection.

While Mom was sleeping, I took the first shift to get my breakfast and get out of a room I still remember in my nightmares. I came back to sit by her bed as Dad left to breathe fresh air and get his own breakfast. His face was porous and long, with ruffled hair and a dirty shirt. He couldn't have slept more than an hour. I squeezed his hand tight before he left to stretch his legs and regain his sanity.

Mom woke up as I was sitting next to her bed. She smiled at me, and patted my hand. "Good morning, Mother," I said in a hopeful tone. "Did you sleep well?" I asked the question knowing the answer to the first four hours of the night, but I had slept since then and hoped she had too.

She nodded her head yes and gave me a large smile. She tried to say something, and I read her lips to understand "I had good dreams."

Another side effect of the medication, perhaps just of the situation, was that she had been having nightmares, dreaming of suffocating in multiple ways since her body was no longer able to sustain its own breath. Good dreams were a blessing. "What did you dream about?"

The question was complicated, and when she mouthed to me her response, I had no idea what she was trying to tell me. Mom seemed rather awake and alert, so when I couldn't understand her, I put pen and a paper in her hand. Her wrist moved up and down in ragged, quick jerks, but she wrote letters that she had known all along but forgotten between full doses of sedation.

I took the piece of paper gently from her hand, and held it in front of my eyes, twisting it to decipher the words. "Dreams" was easy enough to make out given the context of our conversation. There was a two letter word in the middle that I took to be 'of' or 'it,' then I saw an uppercase 'D' and few small loops, and then a tall loop that she went back to cross as a 'T.' I smiled in recognition. "You dream of Dustin? Mom, that's beautiful." Tears gushed from my eyes. During the scariest night of my life, Mom cherished a dream about her deceased son that made her smile.

Her smiled turned into a frown when she saw my tears. She motioned me to come to her face. Holding the paper in my hand, I rose from my chair and leaned in. She put her hand, monitor and all, on the back of my neck, pulled my ear to her lips, and breathed out in a pattern I knew to mean "I love you." She pulled my cheek to her face and kissed me with her dry cracked lips, comforting me as I stood there ready to live the rest of my natural life and she had less than twenty-four hours. I kissed her cheek and nuzzled into her face, trying to hold back the tears.

She patted my shoulder, and I gave her space to look into her eyes. Mom was remarkably capable that morning. Dad had told me she was most alert in the mornings before all the medicines would be injected for the day, but I was rarely in her room when she awoke. She made a fist with her right hand and moved it up and down as if she were a runner, then she made her fist jump up, even moving her shoulders with the motion. She mouthed my brother's name.

"You dreamed of Dustin running and jumping?" She smiled broadly at me then continued making hand motions. This time she moved her knuckle from her right side over to her left, twisting her knuckle back and forth as if pouring water. I shrugged my shoulder and she repeated the same motion again, moving about two inches lower to indicate a new area. I asked her what that motion meant; she said something I couldn't understand, as I was unable to read her weakened cracked lips for more than a word or two.

I handed her the paper and pen again, and with scratchy handwriting she wrote "Waters the garden." I read the words back to her and asked, "So Dustin waters the gardens in heaven, huh?" She nodded yes and smiled.

My mother was hearing her Maker; she was being called home. She knew she wanted to fly away to God's celestial shores, and she had faith that she would be greeted there by her son and water the gardens of heaven with him. Her body may have been in pain, but, with her ability to think improved by the lack of sedation, she wasn't afraid. She was ready.

She wanted to help her mother be ready; she had told her sister and her brother, her daughter and her husband. She did not fear death; instead she welcomed it as the gateway to her God and Savior after her earthly body had failed her. She had lived a good life, raised me with every benefit I would need and more, lived a life of married devotion, and had done what God had sent her to do. She didn't fight tooth and nail to hold onto life's earthly pleasures, cling to her possessions, or desire more time than was built into her genetics. Without the sedation, she dreamed of what waited for her. She was ready to be rid of the machine that tethered her to a failing body trapped on a hospital bed as her son ran and jumped in heaven. Bless the glory that was my mother's faith, because she not only gave me life but also gave me a new perspective.

***

I awoke the morning Mom would die after a bleary night of little sleep. My mat was no more comfortable than the night before, but

Mom slept better without any effects of delirium. She was going to face the dawn as fully aware as her body would allow.

What do we do when we know a life is at its end? How does it feel to know you are bound for heaven and that your body has no chance of sustaining life without a machine? How would I raise a son when my mother had died when he was three months old? How was I going to face the morning my mother might take her last breath? She deserved to go, be released, meet her savior, and dance with her son. I thought I deserved my mother helping me raise my son, but it's a fact of life on earth that we don't get all we think we deserve. My mother needed it more.

God was calling – who was I to wish any different than my mother when she wanted to fly away home? It was right. She knew what she wanted. It should go forward. I would be okay, I could raise Eli without her, and I had to be strong. This is what I told myself as I rose from the mat, resting the weight of my body on my trembling right arm.

Would Mom be scared? She knew she wanted to fly away; she had said she was ready multiple times. The pain in her body must have been immense. Waking up in a hospital with delirium and no easy memories would have been tortuous. She believed her son waited for her in an afterlife of joy. While her body had failed, her faith had grown more resolute. God may not have granted the strength to her body to live on forever, but Jesus had made the ultimate sacrifice to save her soul. Would she stand confidently on Redemption's Hill and let the machines stop? Would she fear the suffocating feeling of not being able to breathe? Would it hurt? Would she be able to talk with me? Would she live past the day?

That morning Daniel and Dad joined me at Mom's bedside as I held Eli in my arms. The doctor was scheduled to come in early to ensure proper removal of the tracheotomy tube.

Would Dad cry? Would Daniel? Would Eli feel the emotions in the room? Would he remember this moment? Would my son remember my mother?

The nurse came in. She smiled. She asked my mother if she were ready for this big day. Mom greeted her pleasantly, then immediately pointed to the tube sticking out of her neck. She tugged at the gauze between her skin and the tube. She mouthed "off."

The nurse tilted her head and pulled her lips back into a half-smile, half-apology. "I'm sorry, Jody. I'm not the one that can pull that out. The doctor will be here soon." She paused and looked Dad in the eye. "You know what you want, though, and you'll be free soon enough."

Dad had been there many days, many nights. The nursing staff may have wished he would go sleep in his own bed at times, but they admired his dedication. These moments were almost as much about him as they were Mom.

He sat slouched over with both hands under his chin and resting on his knees. He hadn't shaved in days; his whiskers grew in grey. His hair was bedraggled, uncombed, and unimportant. His cheeks hung heavily on his weary face. Dad had aged, too, since Mom came into the hospital.

What would it feel like to sit next to my husband if he were lying in hospital bed after more than thirty years of marriage? What would my father do after today? How would he spend his time? What would he find to live for after taking care of and losing his son and then taking care of and losing his wife? What is left after you are asked if removing life support is the right choice for your spouse? What did it feel like to hold the hand of the most important person in your life and know that today was her last day?

I shifted Eli over to rest more on my hip. I reached out for Mom's hand. I slid my fingers between hers. She squeezed. She looked at me. She smiled. I told her I loved her. She mouthed "I love you" back.

How would I know Eli was ready for solid food? Who was going to comfort me when Eli wouldn't sleep at three in the morning and I needed my mother? What was it like to send a child to his first day of school? My heart raced; stress rose through my neck. I swallowed it down. I tugged Eli closer to my chest. My mind began to recite a poem I've had memorized since age sixteen, shortly after Dustin died. I recite the poem in my head when I have to wash my hands for two minutes. I recited this poem when I was nervous before batting in softball. During labor with Eli, I recited this poem to relax: "A Psalm of Life" by Henry Wadsworth Longfellow.

***

Tell me not, in mournful numbers,
Life is but an empty dream!
For the soul is dead that slumbers,
And things are not what they seem.
Life is real! Life is earnest! And the grave is not its goal.

***

What was life's goal? What were we doing here in my mother's hospital room? Were we freeing ourselves of the worst electronic burden? Allowing our normal lives to progress by putting my mother in the grave? Why was I so confident in telling others that my mother was ready to die? Was I ready to let her die?

***

Dust thou art, to dust returnest,
Was not spoken of the soul.

***

Mom was going home to heaven. Her body would die; without machines it would already have been dead. Mom dreamed of heaven, of her son watering the gardens. She was not afraid. She did not fear death. She stood at the door, ready to welcome in death as a release from the earthly prison her weakened body had become.

***

Not enjoyment, and not sorrow,
Is our destined end or way;
But to act, that each to-morrow
Find us farther than to-day.

***

Mom's tomorrows were no more. She wasn't going to get farther than she was today. Her body would no longer get stronger. Unless—unless there were a miracle once the ventilator were removed, unless her body remembered how good it felt to take her own breath and her spirit surged strength into her lungs and pumped breath into a body that suddenly remembered how to function.

***

Art is long, and Time is fleeting,
And our hearts, though stout and brave,
Still, like muffled drums, are beating
Funeral marches to the grave.

***

A miracle? I shouldn't expect a miracle. A miracle could have come a month ago, last night, or at Mom's birth. Why would this day be any different? Her weakness was written into her genetic code. God had made her this way. It was not so tragic to die in the way God made us. Was it?

***

In the world's broad field of battle,
In the bivouac of Life,
Be not like dumb, driven cattle!
Be a hero in the strife.

***

My mother -- had she been moved along like cattle? Was it life at all to live through delirium, sedative, and pain medication? She had broken through it – she had told me she wanted to fly away. She had told her mother. She had mustered the courage to sing a song of faith to her family. She knew what faced her. She did not go like a cow to the slaughter; she came as a daughter summoned to her Father with a dream of her son dancing in heaven. She had been ransomed by her Savior; the Lamb had overcome. She did not face death like a cow. She stood aware, with her family, knowing where she was going, trusting in heaven and her faith's reward.

***

Trust no Future, howe'er Pleasant!
Let the dead Past bury its dead.
Act, -- act in the living Present!
Heart within, and God o'erhead!

***

My mother was still here in the present moment. I squeezed her hand. I had this time.

I held my son. I would remember my mother. She had given me life. She had taught me how to read, held me as I cried, been there on my wedding day, and welcomed Eli into the world hours after his birth. The future may be feared; it would be scary without my mother. It would be better, too, once she was gone; we could heal, move forward, and raise Eli without going to a long-term intensive care unit three times a week. Life had many unknowns; the future was a head swirl of chaos, guaranteed pain, and a time of mourning, but this moment – I still had this moment. My mother was here. She was alive. She was awake. She was alert.

The doctor came in. He smiled. He seemed pleasant. I'm not sure I had ever met him before. I don't remember his face. Mom looked so relieved to see him. She melted into his smile. Dad leaned in to absorb the doctor's words. The doctor checked all the vital signs, pulled the remaining monitor from her finger, and asked if we were ready.

***

Lives of great men all remind us
We can make our lives sublime,
And, departing, leave behind us
Footprints on the sands of time.

***

My son began to mouth at my shirt. My husband joked in a light hearted voice, "I think I'm ready, but my son seems hungry."

"Do you want me to step out of the room so you can feed him?" The doctor asked politely.

I squirmed a bit, squeezed Mom's hand, then released it to grab the nursing pillow from behind my chair. "I'll just feed him here, if you don't mind. I don't want to make my mother wait any longer."

The doctor nodded his head.

I looked into Eli's eyes, stared in the mystery of a young life just beginning, dependent on his mother in every day of his life. I wiped my finger along his hairline, traced the curve of his cheek gently, and then pressed my thumb to his lip, which he instinctively tried to suck. I positioned him on his pillow and led him to feed. As my body rushed milk out to nourish my son, I felt the calm of doing what I was made to do. Feeding my son made the questions stop. Oxytocin rushed through my body. My head felt light with joy; my heart felt at peace. I felt needed, wanted, and comfortable – life would go on.

***

Footprints, that perhaps another,
Sailing o'er life's solemn main,
A forlorn and shipwrecked brother,
Seeing, shall take heart again.

***

My mother faced death with courage and still gave me her unwavering love. I too could face life with courage. I could love my child as my mother loved me. I could nourish my son with the milk of life as my mother prepared to take her last breath. Jo Lyn looked at Randy. She told him she loved him. He said he would love her forever, that he would never forget her, that she was the best wife he ever could have had, and that he'd never replace her.

***

Let us, then, be up and doing,
With a heart for any fate;
Still achieving, still pursuing,
Learn to labor and to wait.

***

The doctor had finished unattaching all the tubes, standing next to the ventilator machine. He unstrapped the Velcro around my mother's neck that was holding the ventilator in place to provide her breath. "Do you want to take this out, or should I?"

Mom raised both her hands to her neck. With an emphatic finality, she ripped that tube from her throat and threw it off to the side. She smiled the proudest, most glorious smile I had seen on her in years. She looked at me, passed her eyes over Eli, looked at Daniel, rested her eyes on my father, then shut them, still smiling as she drifted off to meet her Maker.

***

Still achieving, still pursuing,
Learn to labor and to wait.

***

The interval between her breaths slowly became longer. Her chest movement diminished. Dad held her hand the entire time, sometimes saying her name, sometimes saying he loved her, sometimes crying. I nursed my son, filled with the odd ethereal satisfaction of a mother feeding her newborn child. We sat there, watching Mom rest peacefully. The minutes passed with tension rising between her ever more shallow breaths.

I shifted Eli to my other side. I reached out to hold Mom's hand. Ice. So it was done.

"She's gone to water the gardens. I bet right now she's running and jumping with Dustin."

My father sobbed into his burly knuckles. "It went too fast. It all went so fast."

It was my aunt Karla who called the nurse in.

Chapter 15
Beyond Willpower

As a young girl, my constant goal was to help my brother Dustin walk. Dustin's limits were hard to gauge because he constantly surpassed expectations. He was born with congenital myotonic muscular dystrophy and expected to die; then his life expectancy was three months and then three years. Instead, he gained strength and capabilities until age thirteen, when he had a simple cold and just did not wake up from his nap. His body became too much for the largest muscle in his body, the heart.

While Dustin was alive, I threw quarters in wells, prayed every night, and practiced with him every day after he had surgery and got corrective braces. I would stretch my brother's legs, rotate his ankles, do resistance exercises, and help him practice standing. At age twelve, I thought willpower was so strong that, through perseverance and dedication, I could will my brother to walk.

Three years older than my brother, I grew up doing adult caretaking tasks. Through the years, I would change thousands of diapers, brush Dustin's teeth, lift him into bed, administer nebulizer treatments, clean his feeding tube, watch him when both my parents had to work, bathe him, unload his wheelchair from the bus, and play with him. Most things I did for my brother were helpful, but at times, with my conceptions about willpower and Dustin walking, I pushed my brother past his comfort level and caused more pain than progress. For me, being the healthy sibling, willpower was a tool to push past obstacles. However, the same view I took of my young healthy body proved detrimental to my brother's and caused him pain.

For a while after Dustin died, I lived a pretty normal life. I went to college, dated my future husband, and wrote about my brother. Before getting married, I had a genetic test for myotonic dystrophy, which came back negative. I was going to have the chance to raise a normal family — a chance my mother only thought she had.

I knew my mother, Jo Lyn, also had myotonic muscular dystrophy. I knew that when she shook someone's hand she couldn't fully release her grip unassisted. I knew that for the last ten or so years of her life, she couldn't open jars. I knew she walked more slowly, her leg swelled, her endurance shortened, and one day she would need a wheelchair. I knew she enjoyed her job at Wal-Mart — until she switched stations, no longer had a chair, and had to stand during long hours on the job. I thought she quit because she wasn't tough, maybe even lazy, or because she didn't speak up well enough to get a chair. I worried about getting new basketball shoes when my mother no longer worked because her legs hurt too much.

She'd come to softball games and not be able to climb the bleachers, so she'd bring a lawn chair and sit away from the other parents. Once, when she tried to work again, she fell asleep as a paraprofessional in a grade school class and never got called back.

As a teacher, I tried to be gentle with my mom, but I told her she'd have to will herself to pay attention, try to find ways to stay awake, and prepare better by getting more sleep. There were a lot of times I thought my mom wasn't trying hard enough, was too concerned about resting, or that she should choose not to be so sad.

My brother Dustin had an obvious terminal disease. I was told before I met him that I would live longer than him. I knew to cherish every day with my brother and that, as his healthy sister, it was naturally my job to help take care of him.

My mother was once very capable, beautiful, and vivacious. Her illness crept up in small increments. She was losing muscle strength; I thought a lot of it was mindset and effort, that she could will herself into being the woman who had ridden bikes with me when I was ten. When my mother ended up in the hospital, unable to breathe on her own, I felt blindsided. Mom was going to live with us, help me be a good mother, and watch my son, Eli, while I worked. Looking back, the signs of her disease were obvious, but living through it, I often thought Mom needed to toughen up. I gave advice about perspective and will, choosing pragmatic advice over empathy or true compassion.

The small-town doctor had never heard of her rare disease. When he said, "If she has myotonic dystrophy, I don't know there is much we can do," I knew it wasn't my mother's lack of willpower that put her in the hospital. I had known so much about Dustin's congenital myotonic dystrophy and paid so little attention to my mother's adult-onset form. Myotonic dystrophy can affect mental acuity over time, slurs speech, and creates hypersomnia and apathy — all signs my mother had. There were so many things my mother did that I had wished she could just "change her mind" about. She couldn't just change her mind. Her genetics carried a degenerative muscle disease.

Willpower doesn't change everything. We can't be just anything we want to be. My mother couldn't will herself to be like she was when she was thirty or forty. She couldn't choose to be normal — her muscles were degenerating.

She had the social stigma of seeming weak, lazy, lethargic, apathetic, sad. She chose none of those. She willed none of those. She was limited by her genes, and we were limited by our ignorance.

My lessons from my mother's life are many, but one that stings the most, the one I want to imbue in my heart, is to not judge people negatively by how they act, even if they look normal or have been normal in your past, because you never know what they have to fight inside — something they never chose to have.

The answer to Dustin walking was not willpower. He was not born to walk, and while trying made us better people, more practice wasn't the answer — compassion was. The answer to the feeling that I was losing my mother slowly over the years was not to try to motivate her into a new perspective to magically fix all the problems; it was love.

As painful as some of the moments were, I thank God for my time with my mother while she was on a ventilator in long-term critical care. My heart knew she couldn't get better, I couldn't will it, and all my prayers were "Thy will be done." I took joy in washing her hair and felt honored to comb it.

It took until the end of her life for me to cherish each day with my mother the way I naturally had done with my brother. At the end, I loved my mother simply, without any requests to do better in any way or be more capable. I simply loved that she was there, and she was my mother.

I wish I did that more often in my life. I will do that more often in my life for those who are still here.

Epilogue

Mom passed away September 20, 2011. Her funeral was September 23, the same day her son had died nine years earlier. She was buried ten feet from his grave. Dad has lived with me and Daniel since Mom passed. He takes care of our children while we work. He called Eli his hero many times that first year. He said Eli saved him. My father taking care of my children has been one my biggest blessings.

Daniel and I welcomed Hannah Grace Leech to the family October 23, 2016. There is no one alive I'd rather have watching my children than my father. Dad came with us when we moved to Great Bend. We bought a house where he'd still have a room after Hannah was born!

So much has happened since Mom passed. Writing was a big part of my healing process. *From My Mother* was written through many tears. I pray each night that the story finds the audience that needs it. Rare or terminal disease can be lonely. I have watched how MMD has impacted both the affected and unaffected members of my family. Hopefully this story helps families like mine. It's hard to know what will ever come in a life, but perhaps a reader like me will read this one day and find the wisdom to cherish life for what it is.

What follows is the eulogy I gave at the funeral of Jo Lyn Bartz, the strongest woman I will ever know.

Eulogy for my Mother

Life is beautiful and grand, and the little ironies have a way of teaching us the most. My mother is the strongest woman I will ever know. The strongest woman I will ever know died because her muscles became too weak. That irony tells me true strength is not physical.

My mother's faith, out of all she's given me, is the most wonderful gift a mother could give a child. My mother's faith was the strongest part of the strongest woman I know.

Shortly after my mother passed, we watched home videos as a family. In one, we are at the Great Salt Lake in Utah. The white sand stretched to the shore of a still, expansive lake. My mother sat with her chin resting on her hand and watched me swim in the distance. My father held Dustin. Later, I played king of the hill with my mother as she stands atop a rock and successfully keeps me from getting on with her or pulling her off. In 1998, at age thirty-eight, my mother had a capable body.

If you have met my mother since 2002, you do not know her full story. My brother Dustin passed away this day, September 23, nine years ago. A mother's greatest legacy is her children. If my mother's greatest gift to me was her faith, my mother's greatest gift to the rest of the world was bringing Dustin into it and loving him so much the rest of the world couldn't help but love him too.

My mother and brother died from the same disease – myotonic muscular dystrophy. My brother was born with severe congenital myotonic dystrophy. His case was so rare that university hospitals paid us to bring him in for sleep studies. Myotonic dystrophy affects about one in 8,500 people. In my immediate family, it affected two of four. Myotonic dystrophy took my brother's life and my mother's life. The irony is that, in dying with this disease, my mother and brother taught me how I want to live and what I want to live for.

My brother was the most innocent individual I have met. I believe he saw angels and giggled as they danced. People loved Dustin on sight; all he had to do was drool and grunt, and they were hooked. With Dustin I saw God in normal people and troubling situations. My mother gave me the more typical X chromosome, and I will hopefully live a long and healthy life.

From my mother, my brother inherited myotonic dystrophy, which could be seen as the 'bad' X. However, Dustin's life was beautiful, emphatic, and life-changing for so many that knew him for no more than a day. My mother brought Dustin into the world, and Dustin brought joy, love, and a visible sign of God's mark upon creation.

My mother was not affected from birth by myotonic dystrophy; instead, from age thirty on, my mother's body gradually weakened. At eighteen my mother competed in beauty pageants, and by forty she had one leg that swelled and affected her confidence; by age fifty, in New Mexico a few days before her final trip to the ER, the disease had caused her facial muscles to relax so that her jaw was slack and her eyes were drooping. She didn't have the muscle strength to smile for family pictures.

Looking from the outside, without knowledge of her history, my mother might have appeared lazy or weak-willed. Having been raised by her, watching her care for and bury Dustin and still give her everything to me, and witnessing her faith in the hospital, I know my mother is the strongest woman I will ever meet. Unfortunately, we didn't really know how much the disease was affecting her until she ended up in the ICU at Hays. In the hospital, my mother's condition reminded me to give everyone love and support; you never know what they struggle with that you cannot see.

In the hospital we wrestled with questions about life support. It is a complicated emotion to see your mother cry and try to push away the needle that will stick her when she has been getting stuck four times a day for six weeks. It is unfortunate that my mother died in a hospital, unfortunate her disease caused her lungs to fail; it is beautiful that I got to spend time with my mother in her final days. In her final week, I realized the great faith of the strongest woman I will ever know.

In the hospital my mother was afflicted with pain, afraid of the unknown, affected by memory loss, bruised on her arms from needle pricks, and lonely when we couldn't be there. Such a situation may seem tragic; however, my mother made it gorgeous. Jo Lyn told me she loved me every time she saw me, kissed me on the cheek with a tenderness I will always feel in my heart, and summoned all her strength to wrap her arms around me in a loving embrace. I've always loved and respected my mother, but in the hospital my mother became my hero.

My father was constantly at my mother's side. After seeing my father care for my mother, he too is my hero. My parents had a wonderful marriage, and witnessing my mother wrap her arms around my father from her hospital chair and kiss his lips with the tender gentleness of eternal love made me pray that Daniel and I could have a love as strong as that of my parents when we are fifty.

Knowing her condition, knowing she wasn't getting stronger but instead weaker, my mother consciously chose to face death with her faith and her family. My mother prayed constantly. My mother would ask me to pray. My mother trusted God. My mother trusted God enough to live with the pain, to try to become stronger, and in the end, to wait for her family and show them with firm resolution that God was present in her life and that she was willing to greet Jesus in heaven. My mother requested for my grandmother to sing "I'll Fly Away," telling us that she knew, as the song goes, "Just a few more weary days and then, I'll fly away; To a land where joy shall never end, I'll fly away." My mother let us know she was at peace and would find even greater joy.

The night before the ventilator would be turned off, I feared the pain for my mother, I feared my own weakness in decision, and I feared losing the mother I had had all of my life, the best mother, the dearest person, and a close friend.

My mother reassured me.

The day before, she told me that she had had good dreams; she was at peace. I asked her what she dreamed of, and she wrote she 'dreams of Dustin.' I asked my mother what Dustin was doing, and she used her strength to make physical imitations of running, jumping, and then with a closed fist, lifted her knuckle up and down repeatedly in rows. I asked her what that motion meant; she said something I couldn't understand, as I was unable to read the lips of someone whose muscles weaken every day. I handed her paper and a pen, and with scratchy handwriting she wrote 'waters the garden.' I read the words back to her and asked, "So Dustin waters the gardens in heaven, huh?" She nodded yes and smiled. The irony is that, in my brother being in heaven and my mother dreaming of him before she joins him, I was reminded of the great solace of life: in heaven there is no pain, no disabilities; we all have value, and in heaven we are wrapped in the warm embrace of God's love.

When the morning came, my heart sat in general numbness as my mother slept. My father and I held hands, watching her rest peacefully. She woke up about an hour before the ventilator would be removed. Dad and I held her hand, kissed her, and hugged her, and she smiled. We went through a stack of pictures, reread the notes on the backs, relived memories, thanked her for the good times, and shared a love that will never die.

The doctor came in to ask my mother if she was ready for the ventilator to be turned off. She mouthed yes. The doctor asked if she would like the trach completely removed or capped; my mother responded that she wanted it removed. The machine was turned off, the trach removed, and my mother pulled the strap off her neck. She smiled at us, her burden gone, and drifted gently off to sleep. I watched her breath become more and more shallow, counted the seconds in between. Daniel held Eli, and Eli started to cry in hunger. I let go of my mother's hand, held my baby, and nursed my son. I was feeding Eli as my mother stopped breathing. I was holding my son as the nurse checked for a pulse no longer there. Another of life's ironies: at the moment my mother was dying, my son was growing from my ability to give him a gift as his mother.

My mother had planned to watch Eli in his first year while I worked. She was going to live with us and care for Eli every weekday. My mother and I both looked toward that time with great joy. My mother was going to be able to teach me to be as good of a mother as she was, help me learn what it means to care for your own child. My mother didn't get that chance.

However, in showing me her faith in her final days, by trusting God resolutely, by wanting to see her own mother so much, by dreaming of her own son in heaven, by holding my hand and telling me to take care of myself and love Eli, my mother showed me the full truth of what a great mother does for her children. My mother is not only the strongest person I will ever meet; she is the best mother I could have.

If there is one thing I ask God to give me, it would be the strength to give love to my children in the way I was given love - From My Mother.

Acknowledgements

With gratitude and appreciation, I thank the Salina Arts and Humanities Commission for the Lana Jordan Developing Artist Grant funding. Salina is lucky to have wonderful community support for the arts and many donors who invest in a vibrant community. In particular, Sharon Benson was a source of wisdom as my grant liaison and a source of inspiration in her desire to enrich the lives of others through sharing the arts.

I'd also like to thank Pam McIntyre and the Salina Education Foundation for managing the Jo Lyn Bartz Memorial Scholarship and bringing me home to teach in Salina with the LIFT Loan Scholarship. You brought me back to my roots and helped me establish a scholarship in my mother's name to honor her and carry on her legacy of positive support. So many kind souls in Salina helped us establish the scholarship fund, and I am proud to continue to have recipients named in such a great city full of so many who helped us fundraise for the scholarship.

I was blessed to study under many great educators at Bethany College. Dr. Kristin Van Tassel in particular helped my refine my writing style, explore the intricacies of my writing voice, and helped me believe in my gift. Thank you, Kristin, for educating me as a whole person and believing in me for over eleven years. I owe you for nudging me to apply for the Horizon Grant.

I also thank the Muscular Dystrophy Association, Quest Magazine and the Sibling Leadership Network. Advocacy groups are so important for families like ours!

To my best friend, Michelle Stula – you have been my listening ear and moral voice on many occasions and helped me built the courage to write through the tough parts. Thank you for being an inspiration and a friend who is able to rejuvenate my heart.

I thank all my family members who have supported me in this process. Kathryn, your author photos are an amazing blessing.

Celeste, you read an entire early draft and gave me meaningful reaction from the medical community and nursing perspective. Carolyn and Dale, thank you for welcoming me in your supportive and loving family. Karla, you are a caretaker in the family and have and will continue to help my family through so much. Grandma Jo, thank you for raising the strongest woman I will ever know and for opening your story to me so I could write mine. Donald, Donna, Tanya and my family, thank you for sharing some of the most important moments in my life. And to my Uncle Michael in heaven, thanks for giving my dad such a meaningful job. I have such a wonderful family on all sides!

From the bottom of my heart, I thank my husband, Daniel, for not only supporting me in the writing of *From My Mother*, but for being my life companion and carrying me through the hardest days of my life. You are my biggest supporter, and I couldn't have done this without you. I love you. Thanks for the extra hours you spent with the kids while I edited!

And my father, Randy Bartz, for being my rock, the model of a devoted spouse, a caring father, and a grandfather who helps raise my two children. You're my hero, and I appreciate your heart of service and all the sacrifices you've made for your family. Daniel and I are blessed to have your help in raising Eli Ryan and Hannah Grace.

Above all, I thank God for blessing me with the time I shared with Dustin Ryan and Jo Lyn. I haven't learned all my lessons, but I have learned so much by seeing God's grace and the paradox of human weakness as one of humanity's greatest strengths. To God be the glory, and thine will be done in sharing this story of Your work.

Darcy is grateful to be a recipient of the
Lana Jordan Aspiring Artist grant
through the Salina Arts and Humanities Commission.
Thanks to all the donors for helping make this book possible!

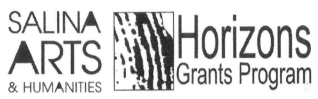

The **HORIZONS GRANTS PROGRAM** of the Salina Arts and
Humanities makes special cultural projects happen in Salina.
HORIZONS MEMBERS are a significant funding arm of this program,
working cooperatively with the City of Salina. These are people
actively committed to developing the cultural potential and scope of
our community.

Bill & Jane Alsop
Brad & Jane Anderson
Mike & Debbie Berkley
Shannon & Jo Buchanan
Caritas Foundation of
  Western Kansas
Paul & Connie Burket
Bill & Ruth Cathcart-Rake
Dale & Beverly Cole
David & Michelle Cooper
John & Debbie Divine
Lou Ann & Tom Dunn
Rob & Kelli Exline
Tex E. & Elizabeth E.
  Fury Fund
Tom & Jane Gates
Randy & Lisa Graham

John & Kristin Gunn
Impress-Ink
Tom & Maggie Hemmer
George & Joan Jerkovich
Gary & Lana Jordan
Paul & Carol Junk
Craig & Brenda King
Charles Livingston
Bob & Rachel Loersch
Ted & Vicky Macy
Gayle & Jane McMillen
Roger & Sissy Morrison
Dusty & Wendy Moshier
Steve & Marty Preston
Research Products
Martha Rhea
Jody & Karl Ryan

Steve & Lynne Ryan
Salina Regional Health Center
Steve & Jeanne Sebree
Boyd & Heather Smith
Larry & Joy Smith
Morrie & Sydney Soderberg
Connie Stevens
Wally Storey & Paula Wright
Sunflower Bank Trust &
  Wealth Management
Alan & Sandy Wedel
Mark & Carolyn Wedel
Gary & Mary Anne Weiner
Brian & Judy Weisel
Tom & Jan Wilson

About the Author

DARCY LEECH was born to a mother whose genetic makeup harbored a hidden muscle disease. The family life was forever shifted when Dustin, Darcy's younger brother, came into the world with congenital myotonic muscular dystrophy, a rare genetic disease. Before meeting her brother, Darcy was told she would live longer than he did and matured quickly as a child living amid medical crisis.

She graduated summa cum laude from Bethany College with majors in English Education and Philosophy, married the love her life and serves as an educator in the middle of the golden wheat fields of Kansas. Darcy is an A.O. Duer National Award winner, published in Quest Magazine, a Lana Jordan Aspiring Artist Grant winner, and serves on the Sibling Leadership Network Communications Committee.

Darcy wrote *From My Mother* to candidly recount the love and struggles being raised with compassion, fortitude and grace by a mother who transmitted a terminal disease to her son and still persevered. Darcy's passion is to use her writing to help families in similar situations to her own.

Darcy is happily raising her two children, Eli and Hannah, with her husband Daniel in Great Bend, Kansas where she lives with her father, Randy Bartz. Find Darcy on Facebook at https://www.facebook.com/darcyleechauthor/, follow her on Twitter at @leechdarcy, see her happenings on Instagram https://www.instagram.com/darcy.leech/ and see more family photos or read her blog at http://darcyleech.com/.

Bibliography

Harper, Peter S. *Myotonic Dystrophy: Major Problems in Neurology.* London; Philadelphia: W.B. Saunders, 1989. Print.

The Holy Bible: New International Version. Grand Rapids, MI: Zondervan, 2005. Print.

Longfellow, Henry Wadsworth. "Psalm of Life." *Henry Wadsworth Longfellow: Selected Works.* Lit2Go Edition. 2000. Web. February 17, 2016.

Maught II, Thomas H. "Science Muscular Disease: Gene Causing Myotonic Dystrophy Discovered." *Los Angeles Times,* 21 Feb. 1992. Web. 18 Feb. 2016.

Wahl, Margaret. "Energy, Dedication, Hope Help Parents of Children with Congenital MMD1." In Focus: Myotonic Muscular Dystrophy. *Quest Magazine,* 9 Apr. 2012. Web. 17 Feb. 2016.

Wahl, Margaret. "In Focus: Myotonic Muscular Dystrophy." In Focus: Myotonic Muscular Dystrophy. *Quest Magazine,* 9 Apr. 2012. Web. 17 Feb. 2016.

Chapter 15, "Beyond Willpower," originally appeared in *Quest Magazine* in October 2013:

Leech, Darcy L. "Beyond Willpower: Caring for a Brother and Mother with MMD." *Quest Magazine* Oct. 2013: 41-43. Print.

Made in the USA
Middletown, DE
02 April 2016